The Bodily Unconscious in Psychoanalytic Technique

The Bodily Unconscious in Psychoanalytic Technique explores how corporeality and body memory can be more strongly integrated into psychoanalytic work.

This book brings together an international range of contributors to consider the bodily unconscious from different theoretical perspectives. Concepts from the work of Freud, Bion, Winnicott, Lacan, Laplanche, and Fonagy are developed with the aim of incorporating body memory into psychoanalytic technique. The contributors consider how severe and complex clinical states, dominated by bodily symptoms and disorganization, can be approached with methods that go beyond classical interpretation. The book includes ten case histories and discussion of key themes including transference and countertransference, feelings of corporeality and bodily sensations, and features clinical material throughout.

The Bodily Unconscious in Psychoanalytic Technique will be essential reading for psychoanalysts and psychoanalytic psychotherapists in practice and training, particularly those interested in somatic approaches.

Sebastian Leikert is a psychoanalyst in Saarbrücken, Germany. He is a training analyst at the German Society for Psychoanalysis, Psychotherapy, Psychosomatics and Depth Psychology (DGPT) and a member of the editorial boards of the *International Journal of Psychoanalysis* and *The Psychoanalytic Quarterly*.

The Bodily Unconscious in Psychoanalytic Technique

Edited by Sebastian Leikert

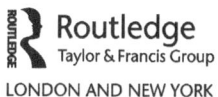

Routledge
Taylor & Francis Group

LONDON AND NEW YORK

Designed cover image: Getty | proxyminder

First published in English 2025
by Routledge
4 Park Square, Milton Park, Abingdon, Oxon OX14 4RN

and by Routledge
605 Third Avenue, New York, NY 10158

Routledge is an imprint of the Taylor & Francis Group, an informa business

Published in German by Brandes & Apsel Verlag, Frankfurt a. M., Germany.
Das körperliche Unbewusste in der psychoanalytischen Behandlungstechnik
(2022)

British Library Cataloguing-in-Publication Data
A catalogue record for this book is available from the British Library

ISBN: 978-1-032-44047-7 (hbk)
ISBN: 978-1-032-44045-3 (pbk)
ISBN: 978-1-003-37013-0 (ebk)

DOI: 10.4324/9781003370130

Typeset in Times New Roman
by MPS Limited, Dehradun

Contents

Translation Acknowledgments

Translation of this book was undertaken by Joseph A. Smith, with the exception of the following chapters:

The translation of Chapter 3, **Body–Mind Dissociation and Transference onto the Body,** by Riccardo Lombardi is by Karen Christenfeld.

The translation of Chapter 9, **Corporeality and Dream-Talk,** by Ewa Kobylinska-Dehe is by Klara Naszkowska.

The translation of Chapter 11, **Mentalized Alterity: Psychodynamic Work with Bodily Countertransference,** by Timo Storck is by the author.

Acknowledgments

Six of the ten authors of this book – Ewa Kobylinska-Dehe, Reinhard Plassmann, Jörg M. Scharff, Timo Storck and Ursula Volz-Boers as well as myself – form a passionate study group that, based on our daily clinical work, has continuously discussed our concepts and experiences for more than 12 years. I am deeply grateful for the highly stimulating debate that has led to this book, but also to an annual symposium where we discuss our ideas with a wider circle of colleagues. My wife, Gundula Steinke, has also been a constant interlocutor for our ideas, but more than that, she has contained much of the tension that the undertaking of editing and translating a complex and bold book has meant for me. I am also grateful for the friendship and respect shown to me in discussion with Lutz Goetzmann, Riccardo Lombardi and Christophe Dejours. They have not only enriched my understanding of aspects of the bodily unconscious, but have also made wonderful contributions to our symposia.

Chapter 1

Introduction

Psychoanalysis and Corporeality – The History of Avoidance

Sebastian Leikert

Psychoanalytic research is currently crossing a border long recognized as such and whose transgression has always been feared – until now. As if it were a taboo violation.

In his *Interpretation of Dreams*, Freud writes the following:

> I am compelled (…) to picture the release of affects as a centrifugal process directed towards the (…) interior of the body and analogous to the processes of motor and secretory. (Freud, 1900, p. 468)

Thus, on the one hand, Freud acknowledges the concurrency and intertwining of affective processes with bodily activation patterns; on the other hand, he feels "compelled" to state this as if demarcating a purely psychic realm from a somatic one. This is confusing: Many psychoanalytic terms, foremost that of "drive," which is based on bodily functions (Freud, 1905, p. 181), already reflect the intertwining of psyche and soma. On the other hand, bodily perceptions are not systematically included in his theoretical and treatment considerations:

> Internal perceptions yield sensations of processes arising in the most diverse and certainly also in the deepest strata of the mental apparatus. Very little is known about these sensations and feelings; those belonging to the pleasure-unpleasure series may still be regarded as the best examples of them. (Freud, 1923, p. 21)

The observations of the authors in this volume paint a different picture: The more closely we learn to listen to our analysands, even where they speak of their bodies, the more we discover an autonomous area in which experiences are organized and stored, and reorganization is pursued. The psyche does not ponder the physical body (*Körper*) to transform it into an experiential body (*Leib*), that is, into a body that is sensed and can express intention. There is no such thing as a purely biological body. That is the reductionist fiction of certain branches of science.

DOI: 10.4324/9781003370130-1

The body is always – and has always been – part of a human relational context that promotes or hinders its maturation. In every fiber of its being, the body is (also) determined by relational constellations. Thus, inasmuch as it incarnates the subject's life history, it is a memory system. The body is always a *psychological entity*: A biological entity whose structures are co-formed by psychic life. On closer inspection, if one must distinguish between the two types of body (*Körper/Leib*), this distinction turns out to be something that emanates from the psychological. Understanding the body (*Körper*) as a purely biological-functional entity, in contrast to the body (*Leib*) as an experiential entity endowed with intention and memory, reveals at second glance that the purely biological body is a fiction based on a defense process. Speaking of the body as a purely biological entity reifies the body, stemming from a defense process that dissociates the relationship between psyche and soma.

Let us consider this reluctance, already found in Freud, to view the interconnectedness of psyche and soma in both theory and practical treatment *pars pro toto*, using the example of another author: Jean Laplanche is relevant to this line of inquiry because he places the body as the primary site of inscription at the center of his General Theory of Seduction (Laplanche, 2017a). In the physical care of the infant, he imagines, the mother inscribes her sexual unconscious in the infant's body. The unconscious messages deposited there then become the core of the infant's unconscious and must be interpreted by the child – which is never quite completely successful. Therefore, the enigmatic message of others, especially the mother's sexual unconscious, remains at the core of the child's unconscious thinking and emerges in dreams and symptoms. According to Laplanche, the unconscious is thus an attempt to interpret the messages inscribed by others in one's body, that is, to transform disquietude and arousal into a symbol, which never fully succeeds. The body as a site of inscription of the primary messages of others occupies a central position in Laplanche's work. Toward the end of his work, Laplanche even reaches the point of presuming situations in which there is a complete failure to translate bodily messages and instead assumes an independent, unsymbolized realm in the unconscious. Thus, he writes:

> Furthermore, given the complete failure [to translate], a place befitting it seems appropriate. Nothing is translated; rather, the original message remains implanted or intromitted in the psychic apparatus. It then forms what one might call "the enclosed unconscious." [...] The enclosed unconscious has no reciprocal relationship with a preconscious. (Laplanche, 2017b, p. 178)

The astonishing thing about Laplanche's reflections is that, on the one hand, such a major psychoanalytic theorist would center his conception on the body and bodily inscriptions, while, on the other hand, failing to present a theory of the body-self to trace what such an inscription might look like – or what treatment technique to apply. To reiterate: Laplanche describes a separate, enclosed unconscious (inconscient *enclavé*) that is neither symbolized nor has an interrelationship with the symbolic unconscious. But where exactly this inscription takes place remains unanswered, much as does the matter of a possible treatment approach for this field. In this volume, we proceed from the assumption that this place is the body and that the body, along with the inscriptions, are accessible through analytic work.

Our Approach

In addition to these considerations, all major authors describe clear approaches illustrating the urgency of elaborating a psychoanalytic theory of the body-self and a treatment technique directed toward it. Best known, of course, is Freud's stipulation that "The ego is first and foremost a bodily ego" (Freud, 1923, p. 26). Similarly, Bion's (2009) notion of the "beta-element" points to a meaningful level beyond the symbolic network of "alpha elements." Winnicott describes personalization, i.e., the basis of the self, as a "dwelling of the psyche in the soma," made possible by the mother (Winnicott, 1972, p. 12).

As a rule, however, especially possible treatment concepts remain fragmentary and fail to provide proper orientation for clinical interventions. This volume contains many works that appreciate the importance of bodily countertransference. Again, there are antecedents. Masud Khan writes about an advanced analysis:

> She cried with her whole body. Inside, I felt the reality of her body bent in pain. She felt she had lost all her strength; I could relate to that, too. It is difficult to put this into words because I felt it in the countertransference with all my physical and mental sensitivity. In this phase, I had to learn to rely more and more on my body, and to use it as a means of perception in the analytic milieu. (Masud Khan, 1977, p. 192)

This makes clear what many authors in this volume elaborate and illustrate through richly detailed vignettes: The specific involvement of the analyst's body is necessary if we are to change bodily anchored states of suffering. Many contributions concentrate on outlining a specific form of working-through that involves both bodies in the room.

Changes in Theory and Technique

Thus, psychoanalytic research faces two tasks: First, to develop a concept of how the body responds to biographical constellations and how events inscribe themselves in the body. It has to come up with ideas about specific forms of representation that the body forms to process and store experiences. Since Bucci's sophisticated research (1997), we have known that bodily coding functions differently than coding through the symbolic formats of image and language that existing psychoanalytic theory has focused on. The second task is to design a treatment technique that addresses this level of representation and enables a stage for it within the analytic relationship.

Before elaborating on these points, let me speculate about the motives that have previously kept psychoanalytic research from moving in this direction.

Motives of Avoidance Behavior

Regression to Medical Thinking

In his work *Inhibition, Symptom, and Anxiety*, Freud writes: "If we go further and enquire into the origin of that anxiety—and of affects in general—we shall be leaving the realm of pure psychology and entering the borderland of physiology" (Freud, 1926, p. 93). Freud apparently experienced the formation of concepts in this borderland as a step backward to medical thinking – from which he dearly wanted to break away to establish psychoanalysis as an independent science. This distinction, however, only ostensibly established the sovereignty of psychoanalysis. In fact, psychoanalysis has always been and remains a borderline science.

For example, as soon as psychoanalysis even ponders the representation of the psychic through language, it necessarily shares its subject matter with linguistics. Lacan (1975) showed how fruitful such an encounter could be for psychoanalysis with a second science that can claim expertise in the specific form of representation. Indeed, psychoanalysis has no home turf: Whether it deals with the physiological ways of the body, with the Gestalt laws of the image, with linguistic structures, or with thoughts on cultural theory, it always encounters other sciences whose concepts it implicitly or explicitly subsumes and incorporates into its object formation. The fact that this often happens surreptitiously does not strengthen psychoanalysis.

Grasping the Language of the Corporeal

A second difficulty involved in including the body in psychoanalytic theory lies in the relative hiddenness of bodily feelings. Body consciousness works as a background function. In healthy mental functioning, undamaged by defensive processes, affectivity, body language, and the experience of moods are core elements of mental events that do not come to the fore. They guide both our experience and our behavior. However, as long as they are connected to the explicit representational systems of image and language without dissociation, for psychotherapeutic treatment, it suffices to refer to the explicit elements of fantasy and verbalization to set change in motion. However, if the connection is destroyed by dissociation, inhibition, separation, or other defensive maneuvers, the therapeutic effect of the treatment becomes limited because many configurations – in the sense of the included unconscious – are not included in the analytic transformation.

Now, one may ask whether the increased research activity regarding the body-self is justified by the ongoing increase in bodily suffering and body dysphoria. I for one would not deny this, and many authors in this volume also refer to this fact. At the same time, however, many contributions criticize the traditional explanatory models, especially those concerning psychosomatic concepts of illness. Thus, it can be said that not only additional disease patterns are motivating research, but also our evolving understanding of theory and practice, which also has repercussions for the best-known clinical pictures.

Contact or No Contact? Working with Corporeality in the Psychoanalytic Setting

Among the motives cited for shying away from dealing with the corporeal is the fear of compromising core elements of psychoanalytic practice. To counter these fears, one must be very clear about the nature of the setting. Beginning with Wilhelm Reich, there have been, and still are, many proposals and experiences for extending the psychoanalytic setting and complementing it with practicing procedures, role-playing, concrete body-touching, *vel simile*. I believe these attempts are problematic and unnecessary, since the intended effects may also be achieved by a technique based on perception. The authors in this volume develop their own theory and treatment techniques within the confines of the traditional analytic setting, regarding both the inner setting of basic concepts such as transference, unconscious, sexuality, etc. and the outer setting. Though this remains centered on the couch setting, treatment in a seated setting would be possible. At no point does this deviate from the established rules of abstinence and the methodological principles of free association and methodological not-knowing.

On the contrary, this orientation along the basic lines of psychoanalytic work is so self-evident that the authors gathered here do not even feel the need to discuss why this decision is maintained. My experience in lectures, however, is that such clarification is important since integrating the bodily aspect into the psychoanalytic treatment technique is accompanied by the fear that one might want to undermine basic psychoanalytic rules.

Clinical experience shows that the path to actively addressing corporeality and effectively including it in the psychoanalytic process of change may lie in the perception and verbalization of bodily feelings on the part of the analysand and the systematic attention of the analyst to their own corporeality. However, actual tactile touch is dispensable because it suffices that the voice of the analyst touches the body-self, the joint attention touches the corporeal, and the resonant sensing of the bodily countertransference affects the body-self of the analysand. Indeed: The authors share the conviction that the psychoanalytic principles of tact and abstinence are especially central to working with bodily constellations because vulnerability and the danger of retraumatization are especially great here.

Range of Indication

For whom, i.e., for which patient group, are the findings reported here relevant? The treatment experiences described in this volume focus primarily on patients faced with cumulative traumas in their primary relationships or the sequelae of trauma in the sense of sexual or violent traumatization, as well as patients with a good or medium level of structure with significant concurrent psychosomatic limitations and symptoms. These overlapping groups certainly do not constitute a small proportion of patients in analytic and in-depth psychotherapy. Thinking ahead, however, it is certainly desirable to extend these insights, experiences, and questions to include working with patients suffering from psychosis, borderline pathologies, addictive disorders, as well as body image and gender dysphoria.

Toward a Theory of the Corporeal Unconscious

To tackle the two above-identified tasks, namely, to develop a theory of the corporeal unconscious and to determine the appropriate treatment techniques, it is only logical to look for authors whose conceptualizations go beyond what has previously been formulated and who seek to grasp the body in its own reality. The authors in this volume all assume, to use Laplanche's term, that there is a separate form of unconscious inscription, an *inconscient enclavé*, and that this unconscious is corporeal. This gives the Freudian proposition that "The ego is first and foremost a bodily ego" a radical touch (Freud, 1923, p. 26). The unconscious is also primarily a bodily entity and is in danger of remaining dissociated through compulsive repetition and a lack of contact with the symbolic unconscious should one fail to establish the connection through an appropriate treatment technique. I am convinced that there is still much conceptual work to be done here and that every author in this volume is making a pioneering contribution to this effort.

Treatment Technique – The Art of the Vignette

This volume's second and equally important emphasis lies in the art of the vignette. My goal was to allow readers to observe the clinical work as clearly as possible, and I am grateful to each and every author for the openness and accuracy with which they describe their clinical work, countertransference feelings, uncertainty, but also the reactions of the analysands and the progress the work made. The risk of being open and forthcoming with one's clinical work is familiar to anyone in the clinical field. But without the fullest and clearest possible account of the phenomena found in clinical work and experiences of countertransference and their development into a concrete intervention – and of tracking the effect of that intervention – this book would have been a head without a body. The development of concepts alone cannot provide sufficient insight into how the individual analyst best handles these treatment principles; without such a description, it would remain unclear what clinical phenomena emerge in the analytic space when one resorts to a particular way of working. The specific atmosphere and the personal and often lovingly accurate description of the psychoanalytic relationship give life and color to the concepts.

Ten Lines of Tradition – Three Polarities

Of course, all ten authors in this volume process the most diverse influences. If one were to assign a specific reference author to each, it would become clear that the ten authors in this volume stand in ten different lines of tradition in psychoanalytic thought. In alphabetical order: Bion, emotion and trauma theory, Fonagy, Freud, Lacan, Laplanche, Lorenzer, Merleau-Ponty, phenomenology, and prenatal psychology. Thus, this volume is not intrinsically committed to any particular psychoanalytic school but rather seeks to map the question of the corporeal within the diversity of psychoanalytic thought. Whatever tradition the reader may be devoted to, in every school, one must first and foremost take the step of recognizing the body as a reality shaped by the individual's life history. Whether the journey begins with Freud, Bion, Laplanche, Lorenzer, or someone else, it is always possible to expand theory and treatment technique, but it requires no small investment in the further development of concepts and the gathering and mapping of treatment experience.

I see no need to present the individual papers here; the authors can speak for themselves. However, it might be useful to point out that each contribution takes a different place in the continuum of the question and assumes different positions relative to the three levels of interplay. Thus, I would like to classify the contributions as follows:

Transference – Countertransference: Some authors emphasize counter-transference as a privileged means of gaining access to the corporeal. In this view, interventions are used primarily to process one's own bodily impulses into reveries and interpretations, or the emotional process is clearly anchored in the therapist's body. Other contributors present their technique such that the analysand directs their attention to their own body, where the process of working-through is anchored. In no case, however, does a one-sidedness occur. This volume contains different accents, but the curative importance of the body-to-body relationship is paramount to every contribution.

Theory – vignette: Originally, I intended to issue a fixed scheme for writing the papers (Introduction – Concept – Vignette – Discussion). My idea was to maintain a high degree of comparability and to allow differences and similarities to emerge. But, of course, this was doomed to fail with such high-quality authors. And the result reinforces the plea for freedom of presentation. The highly individual nature of the contributions documents the respective wealth of experience the psychoanalytic researchers gathered here have accumulated. It characterizes the sovereignty of the research personalities to interpret the set task in highly different and unique ways. Some authors present their commentary on theoretical concepts and their transformation explicitly, whereas others largely accentuate the clinical account, leaving it to the reader to grasp the theoretical lines of reference from hints.

Continuity – Innovation: Some contributions accentuate progress by extending well-known ways of thinking and interpreting through an explicit exploration of their bodily anchoring. Here, the emphasis lies on continuity, emphasizing that traditional authors also thought about the corporeal and that new spaces open up from dissecting these roots in one's own thinking and clinical work. Other authors emphasize the independence and novelty of their concepts of the body and how they work with it. They argue for a distinctly different bodily unconscious and the need to incorporate new forms of intervention into clinical work.

I proudly hand over this volume to the reader, in the conviction that every clinician will find rich stimulation to (re)encounter the body as the vital center of the personality in oneself and others.

References

Bion, W. R. (2009 [1970]): *Aufmerksamkeit und Deutung.* Frankfurt a.M.: Brandes & Apsel, 2nd ed.

Bucci, W. (1997): *Psychoanalysis and Cognitive Science. A Multiple Code Theory.* New York: Guilford.

Freud, S. (1900): The Interpretation of Dreams. SE IV, 1–625.

Freud, S. (1905): Three Essays on the Theory of Sexuality. SE VII, 123–246

Freud, S. (1923): The Ego and the Id. SE XIX, 1–66

Freud, S. (1926): Inhibitions, Symptoms and Anxiety. SE XX, 75–176

Lacan, J. (1975): *Schriften.* Olten: Walter.

Laplanche, J. (2017a [1988]): *Die allgemeine Verführungstheorie und andere Aufsätze.* Frankfurt a.M.: Brandes & Apsel, 2nd ed.

Laplanche, J. (2017b [2003]): *Sexual. Eine im Freud'schen Sinne erweiterte Sexualtheorie.* Gießen: Psychosozial.

Masud Khan, M. (1977): *Selbsterfahrung in der Therapie.* München: Kindler.

Winnicott, D. W. (1972): Basis for Self in Body. *Int J Child Psychotherapy,* 1(1), 7–16.

Chapter 2

The Crack in the Self of Chronic Pain Patients

The Emotional Processes Involved in the Development of Psychosomatic Diseases and the Consequences for Treatment[1]

Reinhard Plassmann

Introduction: Life Thinking Matter

Today, there is a pronounced interest in addressing the physical, the corporeal. Clinically, this attention stems from the fact that bodily also occurs in all clinical pictures psychotherapists treat, though the incorporation of these physical phenomena, both in treatment techniques and in personality models and theories of illness, has been and still remains incomplete.

The reasons for this state of affairs go back quite a while. First, from the very beginning of psychoanalysis as a science, in the context of the conversion model, there was the notion of a "mysterious leap from the psychic to the physical" (Freud, 1895d). Nevertheless, the presumed conversion mechanism could explain only a small portion of the psychosomatic phenomena; they remained mysterious. This metaphor contains the idea of a rather passive body the psychic processes somehow "jump into." With today's knowledge, on the other hand, we can make first corrections to this idea: The physical forms the lifelong basis of the self-process, that is, of the emergence of a personality: The psychic does not "jump" into the body, it emerges from it. Freud's formulation projects a confusing direction: The psychic does not infiltrate the bodily but rather arises from the bodily.

Today, we could thus rephrase his sentence as follows: When does the psychic *return* to the bodily? And when does it do so pathogenically? This approach would be much more in line with what we know today about the self-process, that is, the emergence of personality and consciousness. The mental processes, the formation of representations, and the emotional processes – these are already contained in the earliest bodily processes, albeit largely unconsciously. The body-self and the early forms of the soul contained therein form, one might say, the base of a broad pyramid of unconsciousness, with a tiny top of consciousness. Mentality does not arise by first becoming conscious; rather, the psychic, the spirit, is a component

DOI: 10.4324/9781003370130-2

of all life processes, including the bodily ones. Life organizes itself by forming representations, that is, by beginning to *think*. Life is the stuff of thought.

From Freud's perspective, anything dealing with the body seemed problematic, like a regression to medical thinking – to the preanalytical. Of course, the centrality of emotions as organizers of both the psychic and the physical was long unclear.

Thus, there was and still is a need to further develop both the personality models and the disease models as well as the concepts of treatment techniques in such a way that the body we have (*Körper*) and the body we are (*Leib*)[2] become an integral part of our conception of human life and our work as psychotherapists.

The starting point of our preoccupation with psychosomatic illnesses lies in the following considerations and working hypotheses:

• Do psychosomatic illnesses have an inner core of unprocessed emotions?
• What are the properties of such a postulated emotional core so that psychosomatic illness forms around it? Why do the psychic means of emotion regulation fail to integrate this emotional core so that, in an emergency, the body has to come to the rescue and encapsulate the emotional complexes *ad hoc*?
• How can we therapeutically influence this process, i.e., what treatment options are available to therapists to relieve the body of a task causing its very illness?

Modern Emotion Research

In this regard, it is useful to explore how modern emotion research can help us to understand and treat psychosomatic illness. Today, the scientific preoccupation with this concern is in full swing. Recall such terms as *intersubjectivity, intercorporality*, and *embodiment*. These and many other terms express that the body – perhaps better said: The corporeality of the human being – must be reconceptualized, and that this reconceptualization was enabled (and in a certain way also expedited) by the results of modern emotion research (Box 2.1).

Nevertheless, we still have no comprehensive new model of psychosomatics. Modern emotion research – which proposes the reassessment of the role emotions play in disease and health – has vigorously set in motion ideas of how psychosomatic illnesses arise. This development is still ongoing. As if that were not enough, interest has also emerged in the psychology of the self, that is, in our understanding of how a self is formed, in the sense of "Here I am!" This process is still proceeding, to date uncompleted. Thus, we are simultaneously entering three extensive areas of research: Emotion research, psychosomatics, and the psychology of the self.

Box 2.1   Modern emotion research

- *Therapy research specifically in trauma therapy* (e.g., Beebe & Lachmann, 2004, 2006; Ferro, 2012; Holmes, 2012; Shapiro, 1998).
- *Mentalizing research* (Fonagy et al., 2006)
- *Infant research* (BCPSG, 2014; Emerson, 1996; Stern et al., 2002)
- *Intersubjectivity research* (e.g., Altmeyer & Thomä, 2006; Ferro, 2003)
- *Neurobiology* (e.g., Damasio 2011)
- *Resonance research* (Altmeyer, 2016; Rosa, 2016; Stern et al., 2002)
- *Attachment research* (Bowlby, 2014; Brisch, 2015; Fonagy et al., 2006)
- *Body psychology, organ worlds, transformational model* (Plassmann, 2016a, 2019a)
- *Psychoneuroimmunology* (Schubert, 2018)

Of course, it is nearly impossible to survey the countless studies from neuroscience, infant research, attachment research, mentalization research, and treatment research. However, what is possible is an outline of the basic framework of a model of mental development and psychosomatic illness, the *transformation model*, which considers the level of bodily, sensory, and symbolic representational formation as well as the level of emotions as distinct system levels, each of which has definable properties and interacts with the others. This interaction of emotions and representations explains the basal properties of psychosomatic diseases and disorders of self-development.

While the development of a model to explain the emergence of the self and psychosomatics compatible with basic research is still in the making, we are much further along in the field of modern emotion research. Let us first consider its most important results, i.e., those findings useful to our understanding and actions in therapy sessions and model development (Box 2.2).

Box 2.2   What are emotions? The consequences of modern emotion research

- Emotions are metarepresentations.
- The most important functions are the evaluation and control of bodily, sensory, and cognitive representations and intersubjective communication.
- Emotions are strong energies that require regulation.
- Unregulated emotions cause disturbances in all representational systems.
- Emotion regulation is acquired intersubjectively in childhood and in therapy in moments of secure attachment.

But what are *emotions*? For a long time, in the scientific models of the human psyche, emotions appeared only at the fringe, not at the core; they were considered secondary, descendants of drives and ideas, something that had neither an intelligence of its own nor a vital function. Emotions, as it were, represented the pretty bouquets garnishing the table of events. This view is completely incompatible with the results of basic research and with the meaning of emotions as we perceive them during actual therapy sessions.

Modern emotion research has completely re-evaluated the role of emotions. Today, they are considered the central and indispensable organizers of mental events. In other words, whenever, in the therapy session, we deal with a psychological complex, we find powerful emotions of elementary force in its innermost core. This changed view is called the *emotiocentric turn*. Emotions have come to be recognized as a vital system for evaluating and organizing events, both internal and external. Without this evaluative function, neither humans nor for that matter any living beings could survive. The infinitely manifold processes that occur in the physical organism undergo constant evaluation as to whether they are useful or harmful, whether one's blood pressure, blood sugar, heart rate, oxygen supply to the cells, etc., exhibit dangerous deviations. And that requires evaluation systems that can generate information about existing (or nonexisting) dangers within milliseconds. The results of this evaluation remain largely unconscious; we speak of so-called *protoemotions*. Only when truly serious disturbances arise in the organism demanding immediate action does the protoemotion become conscious and a powerful impulse for action. This would be the case, for example, if a person under water cannot breathe: The lack of oxygen becomes a conscious feeling of suffocation and triggers an imperative impulse to act, pushing aside all other mental content as the person would otherwise suffocate. Yet, most emotions are and remain unconscious, becoming conscious only when conscious thoughts, decisions, and actions are required to ensure survival.

The second elementary and essential truth is that emotions possess not only an evaluative but also a *control function*. Emotional evaluations result in consequences – in one's thinking, behavior, and bodily regulation. This is true for both conscious and unconscious emotions. Therefore, emotions are endowed with the ability to control the energy balance and release the necessary energy, resulting not in small fluctuations of energy distribution but elementary redistribution. The energy released when a person experiences a vital threat takes over the entire mental system, thinking, motor activity, and metabolism as an affect of anger or panic. The same applies – as everyone knows – to the state of infatuation or sexual arousal.

Alas, we are not born with the means to regulate and control such elementary, "nuclear" emotional energies. Rather, this ability develops during the first years of life and continuously expands and improves in later life. Learning to regulate emotions is part of social learning; it requires an adult counterpart with whom one experiences, shares, and regulates emotions in an interactive event. We call this type of relationship *secure attachment*. It is as necessary for a child's proper development as air, warmth, and food are. Disintegrated, traumatically strong emotional complexes get a second chance at regulation and integration in psychotherapy.

In addition to evaluation and control, the third important function of emotions is *communication*. Emotions not only need secure attachment, they also enable it. Human relatedness is based on the emotional communication that occurs during the first months of life, long before language acquisition, and continues throughout one's lifetime.

Posttraumatic Psychosomatic Disorder

Particularly, the treatment of patients with trauma sequelae disorders has provided a decisive impetus to emotion research and our understanding of psychosomatic disorders. The treatment of posttraumatic disorders has clearly shown that these are unprocessed, unregulated emotions of extreme strength that could not be integrated (Plassmann, 2019b). Psychosomatic disorders in the form of muscle pain, for example, are prevalent in drivers who clench the steering wheel with maximum possible muscle tension in the seconds before impact. The same applies to the so-called whiplash injury of the cervical spine, i.e., chronic pain in the neck and throat area following traffic accidents. Doctors then usually search in vain for some evident injury to the cervical spine. The cause may also lie in an emotional shock resulting from violently throwing the head back in a life-threatening situation. The tensions subsequently fail to recede because the affect persists. Here, too, the tension and pain in the cervical spine conserve the emotional response to the traumatic situation. With chronic pain disorders, we also find traumatic situations, especially physical abuse, in the patient's history.

In such traumatic situations, instead of regulating and integrating, the mental system – and indeed the whole organism – resorts to characteristic emergency measures of emotion regulation, such as *dissociation* and *somatization*.

In the former, one creates a sort of "deaf zone" in one's own soul; the person yields all contact with themselves and their emotional life, not wanting to feel what there is to feel precisely *because* they cannot feel it. Of course, this does not make traumatically strong emotions simply go away, any more than one cannot remedy flooding in an apartment by just closing the door and walking off. The benefit of dissociation is that, while the dissociative state is one of emotional impoverishment – and often also one of social impoverishment with withdrawal from entire areas of life – it is nonetheless a state in which functioning in everyday life becomes easier once the traumatic, unprocessed, and disintegrated emotions have been excluded. Van der Kolk et al. (2000) refer to this as the ANP, the "apparently normal personality." Indeed, people can live in this state for years, sometimes decades, often even with complete knowledge that their own inner life is depleted of many vital qualities.

However, the dissociated emotional material eventually pushes through the cracks like the water in the flooded apartment, despite the closed door. Trigger situations in everyday life can cause explosive, uncontrollable emotional collapses at any time, either as a *flashback during the day, a nightmare at night, or a psychosomatic symptom.*

In patients with posttraumatic disorders, one can nearly always observe psychosomatic symptoms in addition to other symptoms. This brings us one important step closer to the questions we posed above about the emotional core of psychosomatic illnesses: Clearly, overly strong affects directly impact bodily functional systems, causing physical disorders to develop under the influence of traumatically strong affects.

Here's an example of physical dysfunction and pain as a consequence of trauma (from Plassmann, 2019b):

The 32-year-old Mr. S. went on a mountain bike tour in the mountains with two female friends. All three were very capable and passionate bikers, technically and physically in top condition. On a steep downhill run, suitable and approved for good riders, Mr. S. was leading the group. The next thing he remembers is his being at the bottom of a ditch, about 6 m below the path level, sitting bewildered on the ground, his bent-up bike next to him, his helmet shattered, with one of his friends struggling to help him up. He found that he could get up and move around and was physically uninjured, which bordered on the miraculous after falling headfirst down a 6-meter, almost vertical slope. He climbed the steep slope, bent his bike back as best he could, and rode on into the valley. The next few days, he did not feel noticeably impaired, but then extreme states of emergency became more frequent; he became nauseous, with violent spinning dizziness, followed immediately by a paralyzing feeling of exhaustion. Subsequent situations involving sensory overload, such as in shopping malls and among groups of people, even working at a computer screen, were accompanied by an increasingly noticeable feeling of panic.

Six months after the accident, he began psychotherapy, on the advice of his doctors. At that time, he was in extraordinarily bad shape: He was chronically severely exhausted, as if doing heavy labor, and in certain trigger situations, he suffered extreme attacks of severe chest pressure, headaches, sweating, dizziness, nausea, and cramps in his forearms.

Further, he felt mentally incapable, completely drained by midday, an invalid.

The therapy sessions demanded the greatest caution and care when addressing the traumatic situation. Every mental and emotional confrontation with this situation immediately triggered an unpleasant tension in his forearms. His body apparently remembered how he had clung to the handlebar grips of his bicycle in the agony of the dive, probably pulling the brake levers with all the muscular strength at his disposal, of course, without success.

These connections between the psychosomatic symptoms of forearm pain, fear of death, and muscle cramps from the nosedive did not immediately become inwardly accessible, though they eventually did in the course of an extensive number of therapy hours. They could then, in many small steps, be resolved by approaching the emotional stress material. For example, it proved helpful to mentally reverse the rapid downward path to the accident into a footpath leading up to the scene of the accident. Such a reversal turns something passively suffered into something actively done and wanted.

In the last sessions of his trauma therapy, the patient himself suggested he would like to mentally recall all the images and feelings of the accident once again, on the one hand, because he now felt confident in doing so and, on the other hand, because it was not yet completely clear to him exactly why he had fallen. Whereas in the initial therapy sessions, any mention of the traumatic situation had led to an alarming increase of stress, now he made this suggestion calmly, without escalating stress, indeed rather almost curiously.

We implemented the suggestion, and he proceeded to peruse the entire accident sequence inwardly and vividly, noting that his images from memory were by now very detailed. He reconstructed that he had probably slipped sideways on a sandy spot and completed his tour of the accident in a calm state, without symptomatology or pain in his arms.

The patient recently wrote to me saying he has since returned to full employment, is doing well, and is also back to athletic cycling again.

The Consequences of Modern Emotion Research for Psychosomatic Disease Models

In trauma sequelae disorders, such as the one described in the vignette above, the connections between extremely strong negative affect and the development of physical dysfunction are readily apparent. This invites us to look closely at the connections between affect and body.

Unlike in trauma sequelae disorders, these connections are not so obvious in classical psychosomatic diseases such as diabetes mellitus, bronchial asthma, and rheumatoid arthritis. The original, unprocessed emotional stress situations usually lie a long time back, often in the earliest childhood, sometimes perhaps even prenatally. For the patients themselves, inner access to the original and present unprocessed emotional stress situations may be impossible: They initially see no connection between physical processes and emotional events. However, precisely this circumstance – that the emotional stress cores are difficult to access both for the patients and the therapists – has led to numerous efforts in the history of psychosomatics to find explanatory models to connect experience, emotion, and symptomatology, that is, to find models of general psychosomatics (Storck, 2016).

Intensive efforts are now underway – stimulated by basic research and not the least by treatment experiences in trauma therapy – to develop new models for developing psychosomatic symptoms compatible with treatment experiences and basic research, with the results of brain research, and with current psychoanalytic models of illness.

These recent models have in common that they approach things in terms of sign theory, systemic theory, constructivist theory, and psychoanalysis (Box 2.3). They can be grouped as *representational models.* These models conceive of the human organism as a complex system with various system levels: The physical, the sensory-perceptual, the linguistic-symbolic, and the emotional. Thus, these models are systemic *and* psychoanalytic in that they assume the existence of a powerful unconscious. Psychoanalysis and basic neurobiological research both postulate that most mental processes occur unconsciously. Also, at the physical system level, too, a large percentage of the events occur unconsciously; the same applies to emotions, which, according to current insights, likewise remain overwhelmingly unconscious. Only a very small part is perceived as conscious feelings. It is well known that the level of consciousness is highest in the symbolic area of language (Damasio, 2000).

Sebastian Leikert's *kinesthetic semantics* distinguishes precisely between beta-elements and beta-engrams. According to his conception, disturbances in the corporeal arise from the fact that normal beta-elements that can be

---

Box 2.3   Newer concepts of general psychosomatics (representational models)

- Integrated medicine (v. Uexküll et al., 2002)
- Embodiment approach (Leuzinger-Bohleber et al., 2013; Tschacher et al., 2017)
- Kinesthetic semantics (Leikert, 2019)
- Multiple-code model (Bucci, 1997)

transformed by the alpha function instead become beta-engrams – which cannot be transformed but are, as it were, frozen (Leikert, 2021). This is true not only for zones in the body but also for the free flow between the levels of representation.

The processes at these system levels are tremendously complex, with each system level subdivided into further subsystems. The more basic a system level is, the more complex and unconscious it is. While we can, for example, still have a decent overview of our thoughts, this does not apply to the processes on the unconscious physical level. The regulatory processes within and between cells, in our body tissues, and in organ systems move in astronomical orders of magnitude. Each individual process must not only be perceived, regulated, and controlled but also coordinated with all other processes occurring within the organism.

The Formation of Representation

We now come to the reasons *why* every known living organism forms representations of everything that happens both inside and outside the organism. Representation formation seems to be a fundamental principle, necessary to all life processes, because it is required to reduce the astronomical amount of individual data. This is done by replacing complex processes and repetitive patterns with a single character. Only through such representation formation do complex processes become controllable, and only through representation formation do they become describable and communicable (Plassmann, 2021).

An everyday example would be a sequence of movements, such as walking down a flight of stairs. Sure-footed movement results from the application of innumerable muscles, the positioning of multiple joints, the information fed from the eyes, the ears, and the sense of balance, all of which flow together as a veritable flood of data within mere milliseconds – and without any conscious attention on our part. Each of these astronomically high numbers of individual processes, which are moreover modified within just fractions of a second while we move, must become *information*. Things in themselves do not contain information; rather, the organism actively generates information. Such information – the Latin *informare* literally means to bring into form – turns the events into a sign, a representation, each of which can then be combined to form higher-order representations defining ever more complex processes for the purpose of both controlling and communicating. We do not *have* reality; we only have its images, these representations (v. Uexküll et al., 2002).

The systems that generate representations can be thought of as layered, building on each other, as it were; in the course of evolution, they arose in succession (Figure 2.1).

Even the simplest living organism, say, a unicellular organism, must have representations of the processes that occur in its own metabolism – of all the

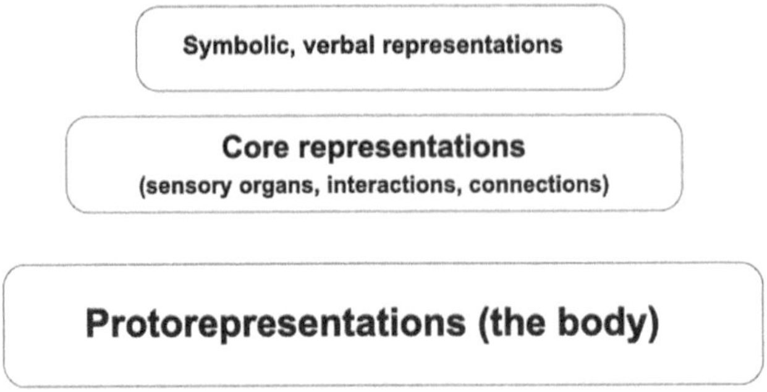

> **Symbolic, verbal representations**

> **Core representations**
> (sensory organs, interactions, connections)

> **Protorepresentations (the body)**

Figure 2.1 Representations as a basis.

systems and subsystems it contains – if it is to control and regulate its own life processes and communicate with its environment. All higher living beings, including humans, can feel at least some of their bodily representations as bodily sensations: They become conscious thereof. Yet, one tends to underestimate the existence and extent of the much larger realm of unconscious bodily representations. Neurobiology and infant research call the representation of one's own body, which emerges earliest in evolution and also in human development, the *proto-area*.

Neurobiology and infant research denote the representation of interactions of the organism with its environment as a *core area*, with the sensory organs providing the greatest contribution to this process as systems that generate representation. They capture information from the environment as well as from their own organism. They create representations from the sensory impressions by very sophisticatedly disassembling them into individual pieces of information, that is, first deconstructing and then reassembling them into what we perceive as images of reality. Our sensory impressions are thus not images but rather constructs from representations.

Conscious (linguistic) thinking, the symbolic realm, was the last representation-generating system to emerge during evolution and human development. Words too are just signs, representations for something else which enable the most complex forms of thinking, deciding, and communicating. This system of representation formation is thus vital to the self-regulation of all systems in the organism, for the communication of all systems with each other, and for intersubjective communication.

Representations and Emotions

But what is the role of emotions in this model? Why do humans and all higher organisms even have emotions? And why did not just one but several

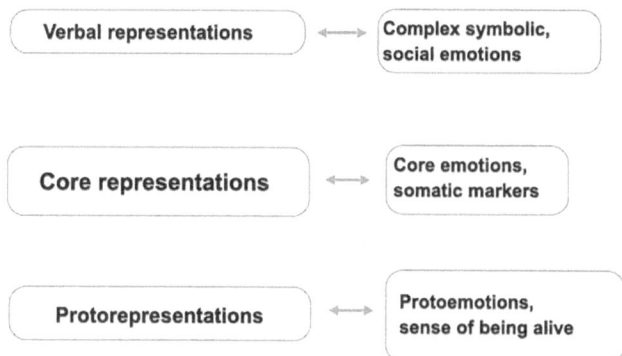

Figure 2.2 How emotions organize representations.

emotional systems develop during evolution for *negative and positive emotions*? Are emotions for us humans nowadays just some animalistic relict, actually superfluous? Would we perhaps be better off without emotions? Will humans in 10,000 years no longer have emotions because they do not need them? And would gaining an understanding of the nature and tasks of emotions truly bring us closer to understanding how psychosomatic diseases arise and how the self develops? (Figure 2.2)

From a rationalistic, logocentric view of humankind, emotions seem to be something like the bouquet of flowers on the table, at best a pretty accessory that adds color to things but is not essential. Modern emotion research, however, has revealed something completely different: The emotional systems are also the centers of *evaluation, control, and communication*. As such, representations are initially only the raw materials used in subsequent processes once the emotional systems have become active. They are necessary to initially evaluate all information according to the two basic existential categories: Good or bad for the self-organization of life processes. The emotional systems carry out this existentially critical evaluation only at the speed required for survival. Any event, say, in traffic, is categorized in a flash as whether it is harmless or threatening. In the first case, there is no emotional reaction at all; in the second case, a violent alarm goes off and a startle reaction occurs with immediate consequences for action.

To trigger such vital immediate reactions, the emotional systems are equipped not only with the ability to evaluate, but also with powerful *control competencies*: They intervene in the attention system, in physical processes, in action and movement patterns, in the energy balance – they control interactions, mental processes, thought processes, and memory storage.

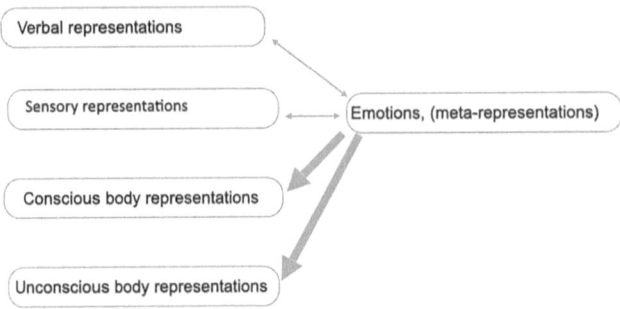

Figure 2.3 The emergence of psychosomatic diseases: Unregulated emotions activate the
level of body representations.

The strong influence of emotions on physical processes remains a normal,
sensible, and useful process as long as the emotions continue in the regulable
range. Only in this range does the process of integration of the experiential
material proceed spontaneously, though it quickly stagnates in the presence
of overexcitation by traumatically strong emotions. And that is where
psychosomatic diseases arise (Figure 2.3).

The emotional core of a psychosomatically pathogenic complex is formed
by negative, unprocessed emotional material of traumatic strength. Above,
we saw that direct parallels exist to the psychosomatic symptoms in patients
with trauma sequelae disorders. When the body gets the task of regulating
affect as an emergency measure, but the body's functional systems completely
fail to successfully perform this task, that leads to severe physical disturbances. In Leikert's words, encapsulated body engrams are formed that tear
apart the integrity of the self. We will see this in the vignette.

The failure of affect regulation leading to an overtaxing of the body
manifests itself in the mental domain, failing to be relieved by this emergency
somatization. The affective slate is not wiped clean and cleared of the
traumatically strong core effects; rather, they often penetrate the feelings and
thoughts of the psychosomatically ill patient with a vengeance. And precisely
because of this intensity, they lead to further emergency maneuvers of
defense: Anxiety states, depressiveness, and nightmares.

The Emergence of the Self

It turns out that emotionally evaluated and ordered representations have
another, equally vital function: All representations contain information on
whether or not what is perceived and depicted belongs to one's self. This
information, which is imprinted like a stamp on everything we experience,
also emerges as an emotion. The healthy individual has a stable sense of what

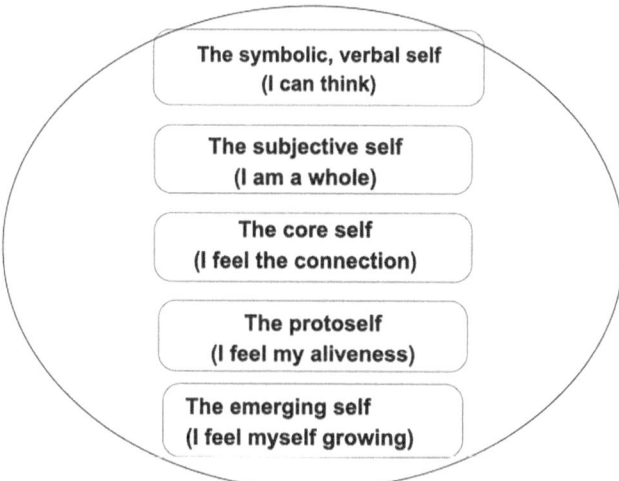

Figure 2.4 The clinical framework of the self, its layers, and what it feels like.

constitutes their self and thus their identity. Yet this ability can be lost in cases of severe mental illness or under the influence of psychedelic drugs.

I propose to call this class of emotions *self-emotions*. They deserve attention because, in clinical experience, they are indispensable for developing an identity and a coherent self.

We have seen that all forms of emotions map, realize, evaluate, and control complex inner and outer processes. And that would seem to be exactly the function of self-emotions as well: To map, feel, evaluate, and communicate what state the self is in, what the inward contact to the self is like, how coherent something feels to the self, and then to use this feeling to protect and support the self.

Clinical experience shows that the construction of a healthy self is impossible without self-emotions. Further, it would also be a biological absurdity if – of all things – the perceptual and control instruments of emotions were dispensed with at this decisive point of psychic growth, seeing that all other processes of life control cannot succeed without emotions.

Neurobiology is aware of this type of emotion, but to date it has neither named it nor researched it separately. In my opinion, it is not primarily the task of the neurosciences but rather that of psychotherapy, which is concerned with the science of emotional growth.

The self emerges in a self-process from all representations occurring in one's organism, in a continuous process from the beginning to the end of life (Damasio, 2011). The perception of the self that emerges from this self-process consists of feelings and awareness for (some of) these feelings. These feelings can be referred to as *self-emotions*, which we can define as the emotional representation of the self and its parts as well as the categorization of whether something belongs to the self. Therefore, the innermost core of the self is an emotion: The feeling that a certain physical or mental event belongs to the self.

Like all emotions, self-emotions become increasingly more complex and more conscious in the development leading from the protoself to the symbolic self. The conscious self that emerges at the symbolic level and in preliminary forms in the core area is certainly the most complex construct of the human mind and serves the necessities of life control, as do all simpler forms of representational formation and emotions.

The feeling one has for one's self is a highly complex construct, composed of innumerable pieces of information on all levels of representation. Yet it is not fragmented but highly integrated. It includes everything presently being experienced, everything from one's history, and everything expected to occur in the future. It enables us to maintain the higher thinking functions necessary to insert events into a meaningful personal history, thus forming an *autobiographical narrative*. It enables us to shift our perspective between the thoughts and attitudes of different people. And it enables us to have a feeling or notion of what is good (and what is not good) for our own mental and physical growth. Thus, the self is a summary representation containing contributions from all representation-generating systems, shown in Figure 2.4 as an enveloping ring (Damasio, 2011; Plassmann, 2021; Stern, 2016).[3]

Treatment Techniques: The Present Moment as a Means of Therapeutic Access to Disintegrated Emotional Material

But how to gain *therapeutic access* to the traumatic, emotional core of psychosomatic illness during a therapy session?

Here, the third primary function of emotions comes into play: *Intersubjective communication*. Through the microanalytic study of infants' interactions with their mothers, psychoanalytic infant research was the first to recognize the development and significance of *present moments* ("nows") (Stern, 2005). Communication between mother and child, and indeed between people in general, always begins with an emotional resonance, giving rise to brief flashes of connection – the present moments. If it goes well, this spawns emotional growth and the *transformation process*.

These insights are also fundamental to the practice of psychotherapy. Understanding and working with psychological events begin with *emotional resonance* (Hoffmann, 1978; Basch, 1983), and *intersubjectivity* (Trevarthen et al., 1998) draws on the capacity for *affective resonance* (Plassmann, 2019b) (Box 2.4).

So, what follows from these findings about the function and functioning of emotional systems, about the importance of emotions for the emergence of psychosomatic illnesses and the emergence of a healthy self?

> **Box 2.4   What are emotions? Working with emotions in therapy: The principle of the present tense**
>
> - *Step 1, Resonance:* The emotional topic enters the therapy session through *present moments* and is perceived by the therapist through *affective resonance.* Contact with the emotional subject requires detailed attention to the emotional, psychosomatic, and linguistic processes (*clarification*).
>
> - *Step 2, Regulation:* Emotions are strong forces that require regulation. Regulation processes are perceived through *process resonance.* Rehabilitating disturbed regulation processes is the main task of psychotherapy.
>
> - *Step 3, Transformation:* Restoring disturbed emotion regulation allows self-organized creative processes of integration and reorganization, i.e., *transformation processes.*
>
> - These three processes, which build on each other, characterize a *secure attachment.*

While traditional models of general psychosomatics tend to emphasize the inability of patients to feel emotions and their alleged impoverished affects (their alexithymia), we feel the emotional content of psychosomatic symptoms is not too weak to be felt; on the contrary, it is too strong to be regulated and integrated, so that the body has been assigned the task of regulating affect without in fact being able to do so. Psychosomatic illnesses can therefore be understood as failed attempts at affect regulation.

This gives birth to the therapeutic task of finding such an access to the emotional core of the psychosomatic illness so that the emotional regulation processes that repeatedly failed, both originally and throughout the illness, are given a second chance in the therapy session – and the hitherto blocked transformation process can begin.

Working with the Present Moment

Access is established through the present moments that occur during the therapy session. They contain the conscious – the felt – part of the affects and the much larger unconscious part of the emotional transference fantasies. The associated emotions enter the session in such present moments. The therapist notices the occurrence of a present moment most clearly in the increase in their own attention: Being touched by something emotionally significant draws attention to the event to when the moment of alertness occurs. Some authors portray these moments as violent, sometimes dramatic (BCPSG, 2014), but they are usually small, almost inconspicuous moments that can easily be overheard. One might argue that such resonant moments of emotional encounter could occur anywhere, in any place, on any topic, and therefore have something arbitrary to them. But that is not the case: The present moment does not contain just *anything* but always something *essential*. For a short, fleeting moment, the currently active theme waits for transformation and further development – and directly addresses the therapist. Such a moment represents the patient's request, the wish that the therapist might perceive a significant emotional theme through affect resonance. The goal: What had never been possible before – achieving affect regulation during the session and reviving previously blocked mental growth processes – can result in transformation processes. Then, the body can surrender all threatening aspects and once again become a normal part of the self.

In the following vignette, the self-emotions of traumatic intensity seem to form the emotional core of a chronic pain disorder. A rupture in the self is not some abstract entity but an existential threat and corruption of the self, perceived with correspondingly elementary violent self-emotions.

Vignette[4]

Mrs. K. had entered therapy because of chronic pain in her cervical spine. She had undergone several intervertebral disc operations, but the pain persisted. She was told that she had exhausted medical treatment, and that further operations were not promising. She could, however, self-medicate with opiates, which she was then prescribed. She had attempted behavioral therapy and in the therapy sessions had been advised to free herself from family entanglements, which she implemented by limiting external physical contact. Yet, the pain did not improve. An unsolved problem remains, she says, namely, her lack of care for her own body. Only now is this slowly beginning to change: To date, she has been trying to pay as little attention as possible to her pain in everyday life, not only because it was unpleasant but also because it contained something emotionally unbearable. Rather, she coped with her chronic pain disorder through denial – a hardly sustainable strategy.

She began the session by reporting that she had recently again developed a cervical blockage that had forced a sick leave and had to be treated by the chiropractor. I noticed in this sequence that something in her description was missing: the pain. She had mentioned only in passing how painful this blockage, the extreme muscle cramps, had been. While I pondered the rather technical description of a physical process, she continued to talk about things that had preoccupied her lately, such as her guilt for so easily and quickly putting herself at the service of others, something she called her "catering mode." She related this to the abuse she had suffered in her childhood and said she suspected she had also been in this mode toward the perpetrator at the time.

These were clever thoughts, and I could follow them all very well, but throughout the session, I got the feeling that something was missing. The patient's thoughts, it occurred to me, had a note of suspension, of incorporeality. She seemed active and concentrated in her descriptions, but my thoughts still wanted to wander. What was I missing? The question began to occupy me, whether perhaps a "catering mode" was ensuring in this session; that I was becoming someone she was serving by producing clever thoughts, by analyzing herself, by lifting terms from my works (which she had read). The image emerged in me of a patient sitting on the train, reading my scientific papers, preparing to accommodate me. Was this an act of abandonment and submission which appeared during the session, at first to me because I took notice of a clever patient who did not talk about her pain? Everything physical – if it came up at all – was largely purged of emotional and subjective aspects, including pain. The patient's body had taken on the character of something mechanical and unfeeling. My thoughts became anxious: I wanted to give her space for something that, until then, had not found space. But what was it?

This sequence in my search for what was missing had the character of a present moment. I was reacting to something that was missing, which drew attention to it – precisely because of its absence. My conviction is that neither cognitive understanding nor consciousness form the beginning of the transformation process, but rather that consciousness and intellect lie at the end of the transformation process. The beginning is marked by a resonance for the emotional that wants to emerge in the session.

So my best guess was that we were dealing here with a burden, perhaps a strain, perhaps some feeling of unwillingness in the context of the session, which revealed itself only in the fact that the patient's body, its pain, and feeling, remained silent and did not become part of the conversation.

Such searching on the therapist's part for what wants to speak but remains silent does not go unnoticed. Patients sense the search process, even if they cannot (yet) articulate it. In any case, I noticed a subtle change in the patient's narratives.

She said she had noticed that strength training gave her a headache every time, but rhythmic walking did not, and she acted on that experience. Now the body, I realized, was moving closer, becoming involved, having its say.

I had the impression that the narration about the different bodily reactions to strength training and rhythmic walking served as a metaphor for processes going on during the session and were addressed to me. I therefore asked whether and when our sessions contained moments like those occurring during competitive sports – or whether, on the other hand, also moments of flow occurred. For example, whether it was possible to perceive when the session was turning toward dealing with traumatic stress material and when it was not.

The patient responded immediately: At the very moment when I spoke about dealing with trauma material, she first experienced an unpleasant tingling in her whole body and then got a lump in her throat. After a short reflection, she added: It was quite clear today that no more stressful materials wanted to enter the session. The spontaneously occurring bodily sensations had, as it were, risen to the top and become a *thought*.

At the end, she summed up this therapy session like this: She was probably beginning to listen to her body. She then added with a smile, "Today, I immediately tried it out."

A tingling sensation, a lump in the throat, and an understanding of what these bodily sensations express emotionally are certainly unspectacular events. But they can be transformative moments in the Here and Now of the therapeutic session: During situations of sadistic abuse in childhood, a rift had formed in the self, but only the body-self retained impressions of the pain, the resistance, the nonwanting, and the self-assertion; for the person to survive, the body-self was torn apart and thrust into the realm of reason and sensation. Here, pain becomes understandable as a sensation that expresses not only an injury to the body but an injury to the self. Thereafter, only the active, efficient body belonged to the self, whereas the body in need of protection did not. Pain, understood as an emotion (Plassmann, 2021), was emotionally so highly charged that, in everyday life, the clinical picture of chronic pain denial emerged. All of this was repeated during the session, albeit with a different goal and a different outcome: The self-protecting, perhaps even the struggling part of the body-self wanted to enter the room and draw attention to itself by first remaining silent in such a way that I caught it – and indeed should have caught it. Then, quietly but still audibly, it made itself known. I suspect these quiet signals – the tingling, the lump in the throat – had exactly the right intensity of emotional content, of physically represented emotion, to be processable: To bring more of what was encapsulated in the body into the open would not have been possible. This small transformative moment represented a means of approaching a silenced part of the self; the crack in her self closed for a small, positive present moment in one place. For this patient, each such moment is associated with an immediate decrease in pain intensity – and not just for her (Plassmann, 2021).

From the many attempts at treatment, the patient is familiar with the urge to try to achieve a lot quickly, always with the goal of eliminating the pain, often with surgery. Other approaches had defined the pain as something she just had to learn to live with because it could not be changed. My approach to understanding the pain as something that belongs to her own emotions was completely new to her, as was the step-wise, careful approach to exploring the emotional core of pain. The patient was repeatedly astonished by the idea of embedding the pain in the events of the session (see above), i.e., of granting the pain a context, a relatedness. Previous practitioners had always seen themselves as responsible for eliminating her pain but not for placing the pain in the dynamics and present moments of the session.

Further, the perception of her own self-emotions and their enormous power was entirely new to the patient, which also developed in many small steps. As a result, not only the feeling for and knowledge of her own self improved, but the sessions themselves changed very concretely over time. For example, such painful conditions in the neck, which occurred only at the beginning of the described session in a rather vague manner and seemed to belong more to the world outside the therapeutic space, now moved squarely into the focus of the session. Whenever they arose or were introduced, they were acknowledged and given their proper space; slowly, the emotional content could be controlled so that the pain condition subsided or dissolved during our sessions.

Conclusion

According to the results of modern emotion research and in accordance with actual treatment experiences, traumatically strong, uncontrollable emotions may lead the patient to take recourse to emergency emotion-processing measures, including the formation of psychosomatic symptoms. The body is then called upon to act as an auxiliary organ of emotion- processing – without being suitable for this purpose. Psychosomatic symptoms can be understood as failed attempts at emotion regulation and transformation. A severe injury to the self – a fissure in the self – can then be felt only as physical pain, as in the vignette presented above (Plassmann, 2021).

The emotional core of a psychosomatic illness becomes re-accessible in the present moments of the therapy session, sometimes through the therapist's physical reactions through *psychosomatic resonance*. The therapeutic process then turns to these present moments and their emotional core, the goal being to address the emotional material in a nontraumatic, processable way: To participate in its regulation and to give space to the transformational processes that spontaneously arise as a result. These processes begin with the emotional resonance in the therapist as counterpart; the emotional regulation process arises through very measured and conscious contact with the emotional material. That allows the actual healing process to commence, during which the rift between the individual levels of representation and layers of the self begins to close. The elements of this process are not linear but rhythmic. One could say that therapists perform like musicians when they listen to the music of the present moment.

Notes

1 Some parts of this text were first published in Plassmann (2019b) and Plassmann (2021), revised and reprinted with kind permission of Psychosozial Verlag, Giessen.
2 This formulation stems from a quote by Helmuth Plessner (2003 [1928]).
3 As always, the poets were quicker than the scientists to see the truth. Franz Kafka (1983) wrote the following about his pulmonary tuberculosis: "My brain could no longer bear the worries and pains imposed on it. It said: 'I give up! But if there is still someone here who cares about the preservation of the whole, let him take some of my burden, then I can go on a little while longer.' Then the lungs spoke up; they didn't have much to lose. These negotiations between brain and lung, which went on without my knowledge, were surely terrible in nature."
4 First published in Plassmann (2021); anonymization was done according to international standards for scientific publications.

References

Altmeyer, M. (2016): *Auf der Suche nach Resonanz*. Stuttgart: Klett-Cotta.

Altmeyer, M. & Thomä, H. (Eds.) (2006): *Die vernetzte Seele. Die intersubjektive Wende in der Psychoanalyse*. Stuttgart: Klett-Cotta, 122–159.

Basch, M. F. (1983): Empathic understanding: A review of the concept and some theoretical considerations. *J Amer Psychoanal Assn*, 31(1), 101–126.

Beebe, B. & Lachmann, F. (2004): *Säuglingsforschung und die Psychotherapie Erwachsener. Wie interaktive Prozesse entstehen und zu Veränderungen führen*. Stuttgart: Klett-Cotta.

Beebe, B. & Lachmann, F. (2006): Die relationale Wende in der Psychoanalyse. Ein dyadischer Systemansatz aus Sicht der Säuglingsforschung. In: Altmeyer, M. & Thomä, H. (Eds.): *Die vernetzte Seele. Die intersubjektive Wende in der Psychoanalyse*. Stuttgart: Klett-Cotta, 122–159.

Boston Changes Process Study Group (BCPSG, 2014): Enactment und das Auftauchen einer neuen Beziehungsorganisation. *Psyche – Z Psychoanal*, 68, 971–996.

Bowlby, J. (1975): *Bindung*. München: Kindler.

Bowlby, J. (1976): *Trennung*. München: Kindler.

Bowlby, J. (1983): *Verlust*. München: Kindler.

Bowlby, J. (2014): *Bindung als sichere Basis*. München: Reinhardt.

Brisch, K. H. (2015): *Bindungsstörungen – Von der Bindungstheorie zur Therapie*. Stuttgart: Klett-Cotta.

Bucci, W. (1997): Symptoms and symbols: A multiple code theory of somatization. *Psychoanal Inq*, 17(2), 151–172.

Damasio, A. (2000): *Ich fühle, also bin ich: Die Entschlüsselung des Bewusstseins*. München: List.

Damasio, A. (2011): *Selbst ist der Mensch*. München: Siedler.

Emerson, W. (1996): *Behandlung von Geburtstraumata bei Säuglingen und Kindern*. Heidelberg: Mattes.

Ferro, A. (2003): *Das bipersonale Feld*. Gießen: Psychosozial.

Ferro, A. (2009): *Psychoanalyse als Erzählkunst und Therapieform*. Gießen: Psychosozial.

Ferro, A. (2012): *Im analytischen Raum. Emotionen, Erzählungen, Transformationen*. Gießen: Psychosozial.

Ferro, A. (2014): Unrepräsentierte psychische Zustände und das Generieren von Bedeutung. *Psyche – Z Psychoanal*, 68, 820–839.

Fonagy, P., Gergely, G., Jurist, E. L. & Target, M. (2006): *Affektregulierung, Mentalisierung und die Entwicklung des Selbst.* Stuttgart: Klett-Cotta.

Freud, S. (1895d): Studies on Hysteria. SE II.

Hoffmann, M. L. (1978): Toward a theory of empathic arousal and development. In: Lewis, M. & Rosenblum, L. A. (Eds.): *The Development of Affect.* New York: Plenum Press.

Holmes, J. (2012): *Sichere Bindung und psychodynamische Therapie.* Stuttgart: Klett-Cotta.

Leikert, S. (2019): *Das sinnliche Selbst. Das Körpergedächtnis in der psychoanalytischen Behandlungstechnik.* Frankfurt a. M.: Brandes & Apsel.

Leikert, S. (2021): Verkapselte Körperengramme und die Traumfunktion – Zur Bearbeitung primärer Abwehrprozesse im Körperselbst. *Forum Psychoanal.* 10. 1007/s00451-021-00425-w

Leuzinger-Bohleber, M., Emde, R. N. & Pfeifer, R. (Eds.) (2013): *Embodiment. Ein innovatives Konzept für Entwicklungsforschung und Psychoanalyse.* Göttingen: Vandenhoeck & Ruprecht.

Plassmann, R. (2010a): *Die Kunst des Lassens. Psychotherapie mit EMDR für Erwachsene und Kinder.* Gießen: Psychosozial.

Plassmann, R. (2010b): Inhaltsdeutung und Prozessdeutung. Prozessorientierte Psychotherapie. *Forum Psychoanal,* 26(2), 105–120.

Plassmann, R. (2019a): Transformative Sprache. Über den Anteil der Sprache am Effekt einer Deutung. *Forum Psychoanal,* 35(1), 5–17.

Plassmann, R. (2019b): *Psychotherapie der Emotionen. Die Bedeutung von Emotionen für Entstehung und Behandlung von Krankheiten.* Gießen: Psychosozial.

Plassmann, R. (2021): *Das gefühlte Selbst. Wie Emotionen seelisches Wachstum organisieren.* Gießen: Psychosozial.

Plessner, H. (2003 [1928]): *Die Stufen des Organischen und der Mensch. Einleitung in die philosophische Anthropologie. Gesammelte Schriften IV.* Frankfurt a. M.: Suhrkamp.

Rosa, H. (2016): *Resonanz – Eine Soziologie der Weltbeziehung.* Berlin: Suhrkamp.

Schubert, C. & Schiepek, G. (2003): Psychoneuroimmunologie und Psychotherapie: Psychosozial induzierte Veränderungen der dynamischen Komplexität von Immunprozessen. In: Schiepek, G. (Eds.): *Neurobiologie der Psychotherapie.* Stuttgart: Schattauer, 485–508.

Shapiro, F. (1998): *EMDR in Aktion. Die Behandlung traumarisierter Menschen.* Paderborn: Junfermann.

Shapiro, F. (1999): *EMDR Eye Movement Desensitization and Reprocessing. Grundlagen & Praxis. Handbuch zur Behandlung traumatisierter Menschen.* Paderborn: Junfermann.

Stern, D. N. (2005): *Der Gegenwartsmoment. Veränderungsprozesse in Psychoanalyse, Psychotherapie und Alltag.* Trans. By E. Vorspohl. Frankfurt a.M.: Brandes & Apsel. 5. Aufl. 2018.

Stern, D. N. (2016): *Die Lebenserfahrung des Säuglings.* Stuttgart: Klett-Cotta.

Stern, D. N. et al. (The Boston Change Process Study Group) (2012): *Veränderungsprozesse. Ein integratives Paradigma.* Trans. by E. Vorspohl. Frankfurt a.M.: Brandes & Apsel. 2nd ed. 2021.

Storck, T. (2016): *Psychoanalyse und Psychosomatik. Die leiblichen Grundlagen der Psychodynamik.* Stuttgart: Kohlhammer.

Trevarthen, C., Aitken, K., Papoudia, D. & Robards, J. (1998): *Children with Autism. Diagnosis and Interventions to Meet Their Needs.* London: Jessica Kingsley.

Tschacher, W. (1997): *Prozessgestalten: Die Anwendung der Selbstorganisationstheorie und der Theorie dynamischer Systeme auf die Probleme der Psychologie.* Göttingen: Hogrefe.

Tschacher, W., Storch, M., Cantieni, B. & Hüther, G. (2017): *Embodiment. Die Wechselwirkung von Körper und Psyche verstehen und nutzen.* Göttingen: Hogrefe.

v. Uexküll, T., Geigges, W. & Plassmann, R. (2002): *Integrierte Medizin.* Stuttgart: Schattauer.

van der Kolk, A., McFarlane, A. & Weisaeth, L. (2000): *Traumatic Stress.* Paderborn: Junfermann.

Chapter 3

Body–Mind Dissociation and Transference onto the Body

Riccardo Lombardi

According to the pre-Socratic philosopher Heraclitus, conflict is the source of everything. Conflict was immortalized by the sculptor Phidias in the metopes of the Parthenon at the dawn of Western civilization: He portrayed conflict between humans and beasts, and the barbarians and the civilized Greeks, or what finally comes down to conflict between the body and the mind. Freud placed conflict at the root of his notion of depth psychology. In our practice today, we are facing new horizons of such a kind that the repressed unconscious is considered together with the unrepressed unconscious and its more pervasive role (Bion, 1970; Lombardi, 2015; Matte Blanco, 1975), with the result that conflict reveals deeper implications regarding, first of all, the body–mind relationship.

Plato, in his dialog Phaedo, expresses a conflictual concept of the body-mind relationship, a potential source of dissociation: "we make the nearest approach to knowledge when we have the least possible intercourse or communion with the body, and are not surfeited with the bodily nature, but keep ourselves pure …" (Phaedo 67 A, quoted by Reale, 1999, p. 209, here translated by Benjamin Jowett). Although Plato's position is not without provocative implications – not least because of his worry about the danger that man may sell his soul for "the gold of pleasure" (Republic, IX, 589, E590A, quoted by Reale, 1999, p. 309) – Plato nonetheless introduces a dissociative supposition between body and mind when he speaks of "keeping ourselves pure" – i.e., separate from the body – and of not being "contaminated" by its nature. This dissociative supposition was to become a constant throughout the history of Western intellectual development.

At its inception, psychoanalysis had a revolutionary view of the individual as grounded in his or her body and its instinctual nature, thus granting the connection with the actual body much more prominence than it was to have later on with the development of object relations theory. Bion provides a lapidary summary of the initial psychoanalytic revolution when he states, "The inescapable bestiality of the human animal is the quality from which our cherished and admired characteristics spring" (1970, pp. 65–66).

DOI: 10.4324/9781003370130-3

The attention paid to reality – that is compromised in the major forms of mental illness such as psychosis – led Freud (1911) to conceive of the organizational role of consciousness in correlation to the sense organs and also of thought as a function with the task of containing motor discharge. In this Freudian model of the origin of consciousness, a principal matrix of physicality, consisting of the sense organs, becomes capable of generating a perceptional flow from inside toward the outside world, and hence mental activity capable of recognizing reality and delaying instinctual gratification, which to some extent reconciles the subject to the exigencies and limitations of reality.

From this same viewpoint of the continuity between the somatic and the psychic, Freud (1915) underlined the need for continuity between the concrete and the abstract, distinguishing between "thing presentation" (Dingvorstellung) and "word presentation" (Wortvorstellung): "When we think in abstractions," he writes, "there is a danger that we may neglect the relations of words to unconscious thing-presentations, and it must be confessed that the expression and content of our philosophizing then begins to acquire an unwelcome resemblance to the mode of operation of schizophrenics" (1915, p. 204). Freud thus maintains that the dissociation of the verbal sign from its thingy matrix can reduce a word to an abstraction shorn of its actual referent, hence confining the "thingy" nature of the world to an independent existence, extraneous and unrelated to representation.

Psychoanalytic practice now involves a much broader range of illnesses than what Freud contemplated in his day, so these hypotheses spanning body and mind can be seen to have a renewed timeliness and a potential for expansion in the context of a new clinical epistemology, which could release psychoanalysis from excessive abstraction and from the awkward straits of a systematic concept and place it at the source of experience. The problem of conflict is now increasingly encountered in extremely radical forms, in which the body and the mind assume absolute roles, excluding each other entirely: When the body–mind conflict becomes intolerable, body–mind dissociation takes the upper hand. A psychoanalysis that takes the most primitive levels of inner integration for granted, concentrating too early on developed mental dynamics and object relations, is in danger of becoming anti-developmental and anti-therapeutic and of turning into another of the many varieties of body–mind dissociation that are characteristic of contemporary life.

Insufficient Maternal Reverie and Loss of Contact with the Body

Freud's theories originated in empirical research: He always defended the experiential basis of his hypotheses, underlining the distinction between scientific theories that are the fruit of empirical research into real data and purely speculative notions. We should not, however, disregard the context in which Freud conducted his investigations, the Vienna of the "finis Austriae," pullulating with positivist yearnings and Late-Romantic affinities. The world we live in today is radically different from Freud's, and so is our phenomenology of mental illness. The agreeable patients who paved the way for Freud's discovery of the unconscious were part of a culture that guaranteed the continuance of the care that is given in the earliest phases of individual development. The modern world, instead, faces us with problems that increasingly express a very primitive complaint, traceable to one's earliest post-natal experiences – marked by the impact between the newborn and maternal reverie – if not actually to the period of intrauterine gestation. The scarcity, deformation, or absence of maternal care has as its result such a distortion of development that it undermines a harmonious body–mind relationship, i.e., what Freud considered the instinctual and affective matrix from which the individual personality springs: A distortion so radical as to involve a dissociation from the body.

When I speak of body–mind dissociation, I mean a situation in which the body in itself continues to exist concretely, but disappears from the mind's horizon, just as the actual baby, originally pure physicality, may not feel accepted onto the horizon of the person looking after it: A reaction that obviously intersects with constitutional factors, so that certain babies are more liable to it than others. Deficient maternal care implies the baby's being required to adapt to external reality at a moment of its development in which it has not yet evolved sufficient resources to reconcile internal instinctual demands with external exigencies. This precocious adaptation causes a distorted development of ego functions (James, 1960; Winnicott, 1958) such that the connection between the perception–consciousness axis and the emotion–instinct axis is particularly disturbed. Given how early this sort of problem appears, it is outside the conscious purview of historic reconstruction that characterizes the traditional psychoanalytic vertex. It requires instead a working through focused on the present, on the heart of the analytic relationship, and on the activation of an awareness of one's own inner mode of functioning.

Bion (1970, p. 71, et seq.) was the first to call attention to the fact that a psychoanalysis that is up to evolving needs a container and a functioning container–contained relationship: A disorganized container–contained relationship makes the ordinary phenomena of psychoanalytic observation impossible, as well as preventing growth and personal development. Even though Bion never formalized a vertex centered on the body–mind relationship and the damage resulting from body–mind dissociation, his hypotheses about the container–contained relationship clearly refer to such a vertex, at a higher level of abstraction. When, for example, Bion (1970, p. 71) asserts that he is not in a position to "observe Mr X because he will not remain 'inside' the analytic situation or even 'within' Mr X himself," he is, without explicitly saying so, focusing on the implications of a body–mind dissociation such that the analysand can seem to be, as it were, not inside himself, or dissociated from the bodily reality that would be able to contain him, and keeping himself similarly outside of or unrelated to the psychoanalytic situation. This brings us back to the importance of the body as the container of subjective experience. The concept of the container likewise refers back to the importance of the setting, so that "the analysis has a location in time and space (...) the hours arranged for the sessions and the four walls of the consulting room" (Bion, 1970, p. 71). If the field of analysis does not have these limits, Bion maintains, all psychoanalytic observations and any development of the analysand will become impossible.

Body–Mind Dissociation, Body–Mind Dialog, and Creativity

If we posit that the reception and the reflection that the mind accords the body form the indispensable starting point of any form of thinking – Damasio (1994) would say that it was only through the body's need for it that the mind arose – then the absence of reference to the actual body inevitably implies the absence of a functioning mind as well. When I speak of body and mind, I do not mean to promote a Cartesian-style body–mind dualism: Instead, I intend to underline the operational divergence effected by the body and the mind in the course of human functioning – what Damasio (1994) calls functional dualism in the context of a position that recognizes a significant continuity between body and mind.

Even if we start from a unitary conception of the human being, we must take note of the existence in psychoanalytic practice of forms of profound dissonance in the body–mind relationship, justifying the term body–mind dissociation, a dissociation that is not about to take the place we are used to recognizing as belonging to the role of the unconscious. At the dawn of psychoanalysis, when Freud and Janet had their controversy about dissociation (cf. Ellenberger, 1970), they were both dealing with much more superficial phenomena than what we face in our practice today.

The conditions we shall seek to describe in the course of this chapter show a distinct tendency toward impasse in analysis because, as we shall see, the preconditions for internal working through, rooted in the body, have been compromised. In addition, the absence of bodily participation can easily lead to the ascendancy of unconscious falsehood (Bion, 1970) or to a condition of pseudo-existence characterized by imitative mechanisms that do not correspond to a solid personality basis. We find ourselves not only in a realm where outright psychopathology holds sway, but also faced with a profound anthropological conflict which is exacerbated by particular aspects of our contemporary world, so that we now feel as if we were taking part in the drama of the replicants in Blade Runner (Blade Runner, Movie by Ridley Scott 1982), who are indistinguishable from us, although they are not human, or as if we lived in the condition shown in Spike Jonze's Her (Her, Movie by

Spike Jonze 2013), where the virtual reality of an OS (Operating System) has taken the place of a flesh and blood partner. Being is under pressure from Seeming, causing an inner tension whereby the Freudian duality of thing presentation and word presentation is in danger of internal fracture and the whole representative system may be replaced by baseless abstractions. The presence of the body then seems relegated to a lost world, in which its needs and instincts are similar to a sort of Jurassic Park (Jurassic Parc, Movie by Steven Spielberg 1993): Simultaneously desired, feared, and denied. The only option left for the denied body may be just going its own way: Rebellion and revenge by means of the violence of psychotic explosions, or the degeneration that takes place when the body resurfaces threateningly with somatic illness.

So we are increasingly faced with the mind's need to discover human limits by means of a direct confrontation with our bodily nature. Both analysand and analyst are called to the challenge of discovering our own tragic conflict of substances, the result of the bodily and mental dichotomy that inhabits us, and to find that each of us is – as Paul Klee sensed at the dawn of the modern movements of the 20th century – "half prisoner and half winged being" (Halb Gefangener und halb Beflügelter): Only the toleration of the sense of powerlessness that comes from letting ourselves down into our bodily nature can give a non-mechanistic sense to our thinking and become a decisive stimulus to life and to personal creativity.

A Shift of Vertex

Assuming the existence of a basic primitive conflict between body and mind, which I shall be describing, together with its various implications, further on, I inevitably find myself shifting away from the standpoint from which Freud regarded it. Whereas the father of psychoanalysis emphasized the instinctual body, which aspires to unbounded gratification, I, by contrast, am inclined to stress a condition of dissociation of the body, or the body's disappearance from the mind's horizon. In contemporary psychoanalytic practice, we are faced with the explosion of an intolerance that asserts itself, first of all, through the blotting out of the body, which is felt to be the prime representative of our limits as human beings. While Freudian vision and psychoanalytic tradition have familiarized us with the absolutization of the instinctual body, we find ourselves ever more often facing dissonant situations in which the mind has made itself independent of the body – fraudulently, of course. Human beings, by structural and existential consti-tution, are placed between the two poles of body and mind: These are conflicting poles that draw us toward body–mind dissociation.

I should like, at this point, to insert a fragment of psychoanalytic experience, so as to begin to illustrate the theme of body–mind dissociation and its working through, a theme that reappears, variously manifested, throughout the chapter. I feel I should point out beforehand that the reader will find, in these clinical examples, a rather different perspective: While in the first part of this chapter, I limited myself essentially to description, in line with an etiological viewpoint – and hence I referred to dysfunctions of the mother–child relationship, which can foster a tendency to have the mind function in the absence of awareness of sensory data – the standpoint changes when we get right into actual analytic practice. In fact, we work with the current consequences of certain early dysfunctions, which have, with the passage of time, settled into a more or less stable personality order, to the point of forming an actual internal system based on organized theories of the mind, life, and relationships. The analyst thus faces the need to consider, first of all, the analysand's working arrangement for relating to him – or herself. This arrangement is regarded as a working one – even when it is prompted by factors that are to a great extent unconscious – so as to emphasize that the analysand is responsible for him – or herself and for the criteria he or she uses. This concept of responsibility as a distinguishing feature of the analytic project is a spur to opening up to change, which the analysand can introduce into the modes and forms of his internal functioning.

Underlining – as we did earlier – the shortcomings to which the analysand has been exposed in his surroundings spotlights the deficit dimension. Without in any way denying this dimension, I would add, indeed even favor, observing the internal arrangements the analysand uses in relating to the body, the mind, and the relations between the two. Thus, we can view the theme of deficit together with that of conflict and the inexhaustible problem of the destructive and constructive pressures to which human beings are subject as basic characteristic elements of human functioning. As I see it, the perpetual to-and-fro from the body to the mind and vice versa is actually the basis of thinking operations. Experience is built up through continual interaction between the body and the mind and between emotion and thought, in the intimate exchange between waves of sensations and the subject's perceptual and mental resources. When the subject chooses to avoid the often arduous work of transforming emotions into thought, he manages only to paralyze his mental functions.

In the context of our hypotheses, the pressure to dissociate from the body should be considered not only in relation to pathological distortions, but also as an expression of an existential conflict that is distinctly characteristic of man and the animal. Indeed, emancipation from the body is an attempt to resolve, however factitiously, the essential conflict between sensation and thought, which is structurally integral to homo sapiens: Just where concreteness and thought tend to establish themselves as independent substances, the human being is faced by his own being, made up of an unhomogeneous medley of the physical and the mental (Garroni, 1992). From this viewpoint, the topic under discussion here should not be considered the expression of a merely episodic defect of thinking (Bion, 1962); instead, it is actually the mind–body conflict, which has profound anthropological and philosophical roots in Western culture (Finelli, 1995).

Slavery of the Body and Bodily Claustrophobia

We shall now turn to a few brief clinical passages taken from the psychoanalytic sessions with Antonio. He was prey to continual anxious thoughts, including the idea that his apartment was being taken away from him, and he felt persecuted in various ways, particularly by the people in his office, from the managers to the secretaries, towards all of whom indiscriminately he adopted a subordinate and servile attitude. He suffered from psychosomatic digestive troubles and had chronic respiratory infections. I feel that the nature of his problems makes him an interesting embodiment, as it were, of our theme.

Antonio begins a session one summer by saying that he is struck by the fact that his analyst is wearing sandals that reveal his bare feet. He is scandalized by the lack of propriety thus manifested. "These are the sandals of a slave!" he comments. He then recounts that on his way to my office, he met someone in a gray business suit with a tie: He thought that that man must also be going to a psychoanalytic session. He adds that it could be his double.

At the start of a session, one is struck by the attention he paid to a body peeking out, thus summoning his scandalized reaction. Antonio himself seemed to introduce the subject of dissociation when he revealed that he had an almost hallucinatory perception of himself in the man in gray business suit, placing his double outside himself. So I might hypothesize that when Antonio set his dissociative mechanisms in motion, he was denying his own physical reality: A physical reality that had to remain hidden from his eyes, disguised under the gray of a business suit, as also under the gray of his feelings and his life. This can explain why the body that the analyst displayed with his uncovered feet was taken as a cause for scandal. We also see from his communication that the presence of his body had become for Antonio like the condition of slavery: Evidently, a condition he was attempting to avoid by means of body–mind dissociation and the blotting out of the body.

More concisely, the theory behind the patient's internal arrangement is the assumption that the body makes slaves of us, whereas he wanted to be free of every form of "slavery," to the extent that he was willing to "do without" his body. This theory, in all its simplicity, can justify the anxieties the analysand reported. If by giving up his body he was giving up his first real home, his anxiety that his home was going to be taken away from him should not come as a surprise: It is just that his anxiety actually referred to his body-home, which he himself was taking away from himself, and not to the loss of his apartment home – a threat which, moreover, he had good reason to know was not about to be fulfilled. We could also hypothesize that his refusal to seek a personal frame of reference in his body contributed significantly to his sense of precariousness as regards external reality: The quest for confirmation of his identity outside himself, instead of the raw fact of his physical nature as the incontestable proof of his existence, led him to seek continuous approval and confirmation from others, from his professional role, and from the advancement of his career. In addition, since he did not refer to an internal bodily referent, he was defenseless before the continual shifting of external referents, doomed to the constant instability that could be caused even by unimportant events, such as a variation in company policy, the transfer of managers or vice managers, or even just secretaries' changes of mood.

We'll have a look now at another excerpt from a session to enlarge our field of vision.

Antonio relates that he was having a conversation with the manager and the assistant manager. The assistant manager failed to understand a reference made by the manager, at which point Antonio let slip an ironic comment, saying "Hello?" as when your interlocutor on the telephone seems not to have heard you, thus underlining his superior's obtuseness. At this point, Antonio went into a state of panic, fearing that he had compromised his career forever. He told me he would rather have been the boxer whose ear Mike Tyson had bitten off a few days earlier than have possibly offended the assistant manager. And he added, "Better to lose an ear than to ruin your career."

I was struck by the fact that the punishment Antonio wanted to inflict on himself for his presumed lack of respect was the amputation of a part of his body, a sense organ, and specifically the organ of hearing, in Italian sentire, which is also the word we use for feeling, both tactile and emotional, and hence it's reminiscent of one's emotional life as well as one's own feelings. So I tried to introduce a comment that might draw his attention to his capacity for internal functioning, which he generally tended to forgo, that is, his capacity to be present, vis-à-vis himself and others, with his physical equipment of sense organs and the attendant emotional resonance (the ear, hearing, feeling). Let's have a look at the dialog that ensued.

Lombardi: You would like not to feel, not to be aware of the hatred that leads you to speak ironically.

Antonio: That sort of comment was out of place.

Lombardi: It wasn't out of place in terms of your feelings. If you recognize your feelings, you can also find an acceptable way of expressing them. As, by the way, with your use of irony, you seem quite able to do.

Antonio: My foot is burning where the sole presses against the inside of the shoe. I'm just about ready to get mad. (Pause) It's odd how I don't feel the pressure of the couch on my calves today. It's as if everything were circulating properly. I feel relaxed.

Lombardi: It's your feelings that are circulating, your hatred that's circulating, when you're willing to accept it and express it. It burns, but not so much as you tend to fear it will. An acceptable burning.

Antonio: I felt imprisoned when you connected the ear with feeling, imprisoned within my body. I prefer to escape from my body; for me it's a prison.

One sees from this sequence of dialog that the analyst's positive evaluation of the analysand's ego resources, which the latter had generally tended to attack just as he did his physical functions (Bion, 1967), had the effect of placing Antonio back within his bodily self. The sensory perceptions that originated with his foot affirmed the existence of his body. And the foot was precisely the part of the body that, in the course of that earlier session, was disdainfully associated with the analyst, who became "a slave." The sensation felt by the foot was a burning, which then opened the door to the perception of hatred. The reuniting of the patient and his body, together with the consequent limitations (the pressure on his sole) and the feelings of hatred, reveal a constructive value: Antonio had the impression that things were circulating well, both internally and externally. Not only could he now discover that he felt relaxed, instead of being prey to panic, but he had lost his habitual sense of being persecuted: The pressure of the couch disappeared together with the sense of pressure conveyed to him by the presence of his analyst, who was usually felt to be yet another of his external persecutors.

At this point in the session, assigning a place for feelings of hatred led to another important perception. Antonio revealed that when he placed himself inside his body, he felt as though he were in prison, a prison from which he would usually escape ("I prefer to escape") by activating an internal mechanism that excluded every form of recognition of his body. Antonio's experience seems highly claustrophobic: Being located within his body was felt to be inseparable from the acceptance of limitation, which Antonio instead erased in order to move toward the undifferentiated condition of limitlessness. This connection of the body with limitation and differentiation particularly emphasizes the continuity that exists between the recognition of the body and thinking functions, which would be unrealizable in the absence of respect for limitation and differentiation.

The tendency toward dissociation from the body, which is experienced as a prison, was actually leading Antonio not to achieve the freedom he would have liked and not to escape from his prison or from "slavery," but only to inflict on himself the very "slavery" he wished to avoid, depriving himself of the sense of identity that comes with belonging to one's own body. By eliminating all reference to his body, he not only failed to elude limitations, but he also found himself subject to external situations that were invested with all the criteria of aggression and intolerance that he regularly set up against himself. The freedom he longed for could thus be actually realized only within the limitations that the body provides: This is confirmed by the sense of well-being, relaxation, and internal circulation that he felt at the end of the session, which we could interpret as the acquisition of freedom that

Antonio was finally experiencing when he was willing to place himself within his physical frame and willing as well to pay the emotional price of the burning hatred that came from recognizing the limits of the human condition.

Antonio's condition commands our attention in part because it lends itself to a generalization that, as we mentioned at the outset, brings us back to certain characteristics of human beings that are particularly relevant to our time, such as a tendency toward dissociation of the mind from the material bodily foundation in which it is located.

Transference onto the Body

"My foot is burning": When Antonio becomes aware of the sensation in his body, he is performing transference onto the body. And just a bit later, this serves to reveal an important experience of bodily claustrophobia: "I felt imprisoned ... for me [the body] is a prison." Antonio generally uses thought in a way that contrasts with the experience of the body, so that thought is not the expression of the progression of body, affects, and thought (Lombardi 2009), but is instead the expression of a state of dissociation, in which, as Freud would have said, words lose their connection with the world of concrete things. To put it another way, the subject tends to use a symbolic system to avoid the experience of sensations, which are feared to be catastrophic and intolerable. In clinical conditions of body–mind dissociation, the activation in analysis of a transference by the analysand onto his own body can stimulate his integrated experience of himself, in which thought can intersect with internal sensations: A condition in which he can discover a point of contact and a possible consonance between his thinking and his feeling.

When we speak of transference in psychoanalysis, we generally mean the transference onto the analyst. The interpretation of this transference is generally regarded as central to psychoanalytic technique, to the point where it is considered evidence of the psychoanalytic authenticity of the working through. Authors like André Green have sought to resist this limitation of the concept of transference to the relationship with the analyst, emphasizing a double transference whereby the transference onto the analyst as an external object coexists with a transference onto the word (Green, 1984, p. 181; 2002, p. 59). This expression refers to the flow of affective traces toward the quest for representations, a flow of feelings at the border of the unconscious directed toward the words of the analysand and the analyst. And in fact, the first time that Freud used the word transference (Übertragung) was in The Interpretation of Dreams (1900), to indicate the transfer of unconscious traces onto the representative material of the day's residues. So Freud had a much broader concept of this word than the restricted sense of transference onto the analyst that it acquired with the subsequent development of psychoanalysis. Significantly, the transference that apparently most interested

Freud, to judge from some clinical evidence, was that onto material that might set up a connection with the unconscious (Pohlen, 2009). And the fact that Freud regarded the unconscious as a sort of relay station between the body and the mind clearly emerges from his letter of 5 June 1917 to Groddeck, in which he declares that the unconscious is the point of connection between body and mind, precisely the missing link that was for a long time sought (Freud-Groddeck, 1973). Hence, it should not come as a surprise that what the analyst finds in his or her search through the material of the analytic session for a link with the body can become a means for the analysand to reach levels in which even the functioning of the unconscious is involved!

In the course of the book, we shall see in various ways how, at primitive levels, a working through constantly focused on the analyst can be anti-developmental and anti-therapeutic, distancing the subject from himself in all those states in which he has trouble relating to his own body and his own primary emotional levels. He is thus exposed to the risk of the paralyzing regressive dynamics of compliance and imitation. When we work with primitive mental states, the transference onto the analyst cohabits with the transference onto the body: Concentrating on the latter as the driving force of the working through makes it possible to construct, in the mid of the analytic session, a fabric of body–mind connections to which the patient would otherwise not have access. Ferrari (1992) conceptualized the contemporaneous progression of the body–mind relationship and the analysand-analyst relationship as a vertical axis and a horizontal axis, respectively. This "vertical" transference of the analysand onto his own body could not take place without a reverie (Bion, 1962) based on the analyst's capacity for "listening" to his own sensory world; thus, there comes about in the session a double and parallel transference on the part of the participants each onto his own corporality. This focus on bodily participation decisively facilitates the processes of empathy and emotional communication within the analytic couple, since a connection with sensations and sensitivity in general is a precondition for the emotional life.

The focus on the transference to the body is of essence, particularly when the analysand shows an absence of emotional resonance, together with clear manifestations of estrangement from or indifference toward himself and his own physicality. I would emphasize that transference onto the body makes it possible to reach a level of experience that cannot necessarily be reduced to terms of particular mental contents. In fact, exploring feeling as a general human category brings up our vaster original condition – which itself cannot be directly reduced to symbolic terms and which is ingrained in our identity as homo sapiens – in which the duality of knowing and feeling coexists with that of mind and body as identity: Our awareness of bodily feeling can be the source of "the very sense of being, which is in continuous opposition to non-sense" (Garroni, 1992, p. 15).

Bodily Countertransference

The primacy of the sensory pressure that comes to light when the working through creates a connection with bodily experience means that the analyst must operate on the same unorganized levels of fluid, untranslatable, and potentially explosive sensations that the analysand is living through. Thus, the patient's bodily pressures – even before they are understood – should be cooled down, principally by means of the resources of internal containment. At these primitive levels, the analyst is confronted not so much with specific mental content or clear-cut conflictual areas, like those one finds in the more integrated phenomena of the countertransference, as instead with more radical and primitive manifestations – which I shall indicate here with the term somatic countertransference – so that the analyst finds himself containing in his own body the pre-symbolic sensory manifestations that predate mental phenomena, thereby fostering the conditions for mental functioning at more evolved levels.

There is now a general agreement to regard the countertransference primarily in its non-pathological and non-refractory aspects. When primitive levels connected with bodily experience are in play, one has experiences that are distinctly characterized by unconscious participation and in which anxiety can easily become oceanic (Freud, 1930). These archaic levels involve approaching non- and pre-symbolic areas marked by indifferentiation and concreteness. In the course of psychoanalysis, the progress of the working through can include confronting extreme phenomena of body–mind dissociation, with the sudden and sometimes long involvement of various sorts of somatic reactions. The somatic countertransference is actually the analyst's transference onto his own body, which is a prerequisite for accompanying the analysand's working through the approach to his own body, particularly in developmental conditions in which the patient's body–mind dissociation is no longer in control. Here one encounters the various sensory sensibilities of analysts, so that one might especially notice Freud's hearing faculty in relation to his patients or the particular visual quality of Melanie Klein's clinical talent. At the most primitive levels, phenomena of more diffuse reactivity enter into play, so the analyst's body functions like a receptor organ for the analysand's unconscious communications. The whole body becomes a sort of tympanic membrane for receiving purposes.

The somatic countertransference can appear in the most varied ways, including a particular sensitivity to internal movements. So certain sense experiences draw the attention of the mind, as if they were subjected to the mediation of a magnifying glass: For instance, the sensory acuity of particular areas of the body and various subjective somatic phenomena such as sensations of heat, nausea, dizziness, changes in respiratory rhythm, etc., as well as transitory physical indispositions (pains, muscular contractions, cardiac arrhythmias, etc.). These somatic phenomena can be accompanied by a transitory limitation of the resources of abstraction: The analyst's cathectic energy directed toward sensory-emotional levels can facilitate a willingness to contain sensory-emotional experience, which is in the process of being organized within the analysand.

A Psychosensory Pentagram

Over the course of time, I have noticed how my analytic listening is greatly conditioned by some of my internal sensory movements, such as the perception of the weight and heat of my body, especially in the lumbar region. My disposition for listening to a patient's communications could not include emotional participation, not to mention rational comprehension, without my personal sensory focusing, from which my affective resonance and my intellectual activity branch out. It forms a sensory background that functions, in organizational terms, as a sort of psychosensory pentagram, on which there gradually gather traces of communication, both emotional and rational, from the analysand.

Considerable attention and dedication are called for in receiving the phenomenon of the so-called somatic countertransference, since physical emotions can be violent and difficult to contain, and their metabolization time must be patiently allowed for. This time is independent of the analyst's will and can enter into conflict with other aspects of his life. The emotional working through of the deeper levels extends, in fact, well beyond the confines of the session and may also exclude the conscious levels: It is hardly an accident that Freud, in his last work (1940), tended to attribute to bodily sensations a close correspondence to unconscious phenomena. The analyst is thus called upon to be aware of his internal reactions even outside his office, bearing in mind that they can perfectly well show up when he least expects them. Well beyond our conscious will, the experience we have with our analysands accompanies us continuously, and the related emotional working through is continuous, active, and intense.

I shall give a brief example of the problems that emerge from the need to respect our sensory-emotional bodily reactions and the specific time their working through requires. The example is taken from a turbulent period of the treatment of one of the cases we shall encounter later in the book. After some very dramatic sessions with personal attacks and many sorts of insults from the patient, I had gotten into the habit of allowing myself time for working through the state of physical chaos in which the end of the session generally left me. I was indeed often completely exhausted, as if I had finished a race or some enormous physical task; my breathing was shallow and labored, and I had palpitations, all in connection with the emotional violence that had emerged during the session. Only some time to rest – as when one catches one's breath after a long run – would bring about a gradual reduction in my somatic reactions and allow me to put my sensory world back in order. One day I had not succeeded in scheduling my dentist's appointment at a more convenient time, and I had to leave my office without my habitual period of emotional decompression after these sessions. I had no time to lose, so I quickly grabbed the removable car radio from my car, but I moved in such haste that the radio fell onto my foot, causing a serious contusion, as a result of which I later had to have the nail of my big toe surgically removed. This trivial episode becomes significant if we consider that, were these forms of loss of motor coordination to increase, they could well cause accidents of far from trifling importance to the analyst. It can perhaps give us an idea of the risks implicit in the micro- and macro-phenomena of body–mind dissociation to which an analyst who works with difficult cases can be exposed and of the caution and care that his self-government requires, going far beyond the specific processes of comprehension that are involved in more developed and mentalized areas. While comprehension can be very swift, emotional digestion takes considerable time, and one must allow the affects to follow their own tempo.

Because of the objective difficulty of describing the involvement of the various levels called upon in clinical experience, I shall not always manage, in the course of the book, to faithfully represent the three-dimensionality of my subjective experience with all its somatic implications. Hence, I leave it to the sensitivity and intuition of the reader to imagine the foreseeable sensory and emotional reactions that accompany the exploration of the most primitive levels of human experience.

Toward a New Centrality of the Analysand

In this book, I propose a radical shift of emphasis, such that the interest in the body is not limited to its symbolic meaning or to related unconscious phantasies. In other words, all of psychoanalysis does not come down to a mere metaphorization – with all due respect to the undeniable value of metaphors – but does instead call for a confrontation with reality, and with that first expression of reality, the body. In many cases, a working through aimed at a relationship with one's own body is the groundwork for mental functioning, offering a concrete referent for what Freud called thing presentation: Thanks to the real referent introduced by the body, this presentation begins to make sense, together with a personal experience of one's own unconscious. In the absence of the concrete internal referent of one's own body, the work done on symbols is in danger of remaining abstractly self-referential, empty of personal substance, and anti-developmental.

In the last few decades, the body–mind relationship has been underestimated in our discipline, probably because it could involve a retrenchment of the interpretative and metaphorizing power of psychoanalysis, since it spotlights elements of evidence that might be felt to diminish the intellectual status of the analyst.

Some analysts are capable of taking as a sort of threat to their identity the increasing importance of concreteness and the limited ability to deal with metaphoric levels in so many people who now enter analysis. In fact, even in patients with apparently developed mentalization, it often happens that the evolution of the analytic process includes a valorization of the more concrete levels of experience, so that a link between thought and the actual physical person of the subject can be constructed.

The real and concrete body has been forgotten in psychoanalysis, perhaps also because it reduces the charismatic power of the psychoanalyst as the "expert" in terms of the analysand's situation: It is not fortuitous that recognizing the existence of an actual body implies the recognition of the real barriers that pertain to bodies, so that the analysand is the only one who can actually be an expert about himself – about what takes place within his own "borders" – and thus the analyst is structurally prevented from going beyond a hypothesis, a suggestion, or an external catalysis of the phenomena that remain substantially internal to and primarily within the province of the analysand. It was with telling perspicacity that Bion noted that patients' problems "are due not to their failure to represent but to their failure to be" (1970, p. 18).

Placing the body in the foreground in psychoanalysis implies giving back to the analysand a territory where he has a genuine expertise and authority: An authority that has too often been overshadowed by an analytic culture that is maddeningly focused on the interpretation of the transference and the request for dependency. Valorizing the body in psychoanalysis can therefore have a decisive protective function in the face of unwitting operations of colonization and subjection of the patient to analytic knowledge. It can also militate against losing awareness of the decisive role of responsibility that the analysand continues to play toward himself, even in the intimately relational context of the analytic process. And I hope that what I have given a preview of in this chapter will become increasingly resonant and intelligible to the reader as he or she proceeds with the reading of the book.

References

Bion, W. R. (1962): *Learning from Experience*. London: Karnac.
Bion, W. R. (1967): Attacks on linking. In: *Second Thoughts*. London: Karnac, 93–110.
Bion, W. R. (1970): *Attention and Interpretation*. London: Tavistock.
Damasio, A. (1994): *Decartes' Error. Emotion, Reason and the Human Brain*. New York: Putnam.
Ellenberger, H. F. (1970): *Discovery of the Unconscious: The History and Evolution of Dynamic Psychiatry*. New York: Basic Books.
Ferrari, A. B. (1992): *L'eclissi del corpo*. Rome: Borla, 7–16.
Finelli, R. (1995): Mente e corpo tra due e tre. *Almanacchi nuovi*, 2/3, 132–139.
Freud, S. (1900): The Interpretation of Dreams. SE IV, 1–625
Freud, S. (1911): Formulations on the two principles of mental functioning. SE X, 218–226.
Freud, S. (1915): *The Unconscious*. SE XXIV, 159–215.

Freud, S. (1930): Civilization and Its Discontents. SE XXI.

Freud, S. (1938): Outline of Psychoanalysis. SE XXIII.

Freud, S. & Groddeck, G. (1973): *Carteggio*. Milano: Adelphi.

Garroni, E. (1992): Che cosa si prova ad essere un *Homo sapiens*? Introduction to A. B.

Green, A. (1984): Le langage dans la psychanalyse. In: *Languages*. Paris: Edition Les Belles Lettres, 19–250.

Green, A. (2002): *La Pensée clinique*. Paris: Edition Odile Jacob.

James, M. (1960): Premature ego development. Some observations on disturbances in the first three months of life. *Int J Psychoanal*, 41, 288–294.

Lombardi, R. (2009): Body, affect, thought: Reflections of the work of Matte Blanco and Ferrari. *Psychoanal Q*, 78, 126–160.

Lombardi, R. (2015): *Formless Infinity. Clinical Explorations of Matte Blanco and Bion*. London (The New Library of Psychoanalysis).

Matte Blanco, I. (1975): *The Unconscious as Infinite Sets*. London: Duckworth.

Pohlen, M. (2009): *In analisi con Freud: I verbali delle sedute di Ernst Blum del 1922*. Turin: Boringhieri.

Reale, G. (1999): *Corpo, anima e salute: Il concetto di uomo da Omero a Platone*. Milan: Cortina.

Winnicott, D. W. (1958): Withdrawl and regression. In: *Through Paediatrics to Psychoanalysis: Collected Papers*. London: Tavistock, 243–254.

Chapter 4

How To Begin?

Jörg M. Scharff

While thinking about a suitable contribution for this volume, I was reminded of the patient whose treatment I report in the following. She was a pretty, subtle, and sensitive middle-aged woman who quickly won my sympathy. What she told me about her private life had a thoughtful and mature effect on me, as did what she told me about her professional environment. She came to me because of contact difficulties, and it was easy to assume that these resulted from an early disturbance in the relationship with her mother.

My remarks focus on how traces of this early tragic incident were enacted in the interpersonal relationship between the patient and me, as revealed by eye contact and some gestures. When I look back on the overall successful course of the weekly 1-hour therapy, I find it difficult to differentiate between a fundamentally new form of relationship that developed during the therapeutic process and the role therapy played in allowing the patient to rediscover what had been positive in her childhood environment by reconnecting with good experiences.

I cannot discuss all the therapeutic actions and omissions that may have been helpful in the therapy. Given the general theme of this book, I rather have selected three factors that, in retrospect, I consider to have been beneficial in some specific way:

1 Being aware of the bodily state – especially of my own – in the space of a session with the patient.[1]
2 Maintaining a physically grounded attitude of patience, which gives space for something that is not (yet) possible (Schneider, 2006, p. 915; Staehle, 2009, pp. 186 f.).
3 Projecting a willingness to make myself available in moments when being directly addressed, more so than is customarily found in such an encounter.

The level at issue here is so "deep" that I hope to be able to share the essentials with the readers while dispensing with further biographical details and details of personal appearance.

DOI: 10.4324/9781003370130-4

Alas, there was no final result whereby all the old patterns disappeared forever; to the very end, it required a constant effort on both sides to recognize the old and give the new a chance. However, the repeated experiences of working through things resulted in an ever more anchored hope that it would be possible to find a common path in situations initially experienced as difficult, in which new possibilities for experiences and relationships would be revealed.

The Stage

The patient usually arrives a few minutes late for the session. As she enters my room, she fixates her gaze on me, occasionally with an almost piercing effect. I experience myself as being exposed to something intrusive approaching me, causing me to clam up involuntarily. Her gaze also seems strangely hardened and rigid, sometimes as if frozen. Is she really trying to catch my eye, or is she in fact looking right through me? It is as if the patient is not reaching out to me and, having approached, is trying to draw me to her. I feel fixated and simultaneously kept at arm's length. I cannot engage with her as a living creature. I feel exposed to something so controlling that it prevents any movement of my own. A rigidity receives me, absent of a searching gaze that might enable us to open ourselves expectantly in an attempt at mutual coordination from the beginning.

Corresponding to the relational event that occurs on the gaze level is a detail in the gestures exchanged during the greeting: The patient, although she holds me apart from her with a slightly stiffened arm, at the same time physically comes just a little too close to me, albeit without relinquishing her hand when we shake hands. Again, this rigid, somewhat clinging grip. Although I experience this gesture as intrusive, it also takes on something inappropriately buddy-like for me. On the verbal level, this corresponds to the camaraderie of a "bye, bye" when the patient leaves.

These scenes expose me to the coexistence of rigidity and intrusion, distance and absence of distance, and oppressive clinginess and dis-engagement. Without any means available to me to influence this state of affairs, my body shuts off. Once this happens, I feel a strange, unwelcome, defensive stiffening in my body, a sign that something in me is resisting what I perceive to be manipulation. I have lost access to my usual ability to react and resonate as a therapist, and I feel dispossessed of myself.

My interaction with the patient now reverts to the usual schematic routine, the only thing I can safely hold on to. I do not look at the patient; rather, alienally and unintentionally, I come to view her from above. Then, when our hands part, we go to our respective places, as if we are both adhering to some regulation: "There's where the patient sits, here's where the therapist sits." My breathing is not free, I feel constricted.

Superficially, the patient has found her way into my treatment room, albeit belatedly. Yet, she lacks an inner expectation of arriving in my presence, of opening up to me. So, the patient is there, but actually *not* there. The welcoming ritual is determined by a compulsively controlling process, whereby the paradoxical goal of this act of appropriation is probably to keep the other at bay. An air of armored autonomy dominates: Nothing seems to be expected of the other. Every form of cautious encounter – in the sense of fine-tuning the interbody event – is blocked in advance. We do not truly come together.

What I am describing here only gradually dawned on me. While writing these words, it seems to me as though the events between us become real only through the words I am now using in my attempt to capture them, but without seeming to me to be an invention. Certainly, at the beginning, I felt the tendency to smooth out what I had experienced, to keep it at the periphery of my consciousness and tick it off, in order to concentrate primarily on what the patient was communicating to me verbally during the session. Something in me resisted perceiving this interaction between us as it had actually occurred. But perhaps, at the time, I had no other choice because otherwise I would have been completely overwhelmed by not knowing which way to turn.

She says:

"When you speak, I am quite surprised you are there."

"Between sessions, I don't miss you. You're just, you know, gone. When I come to you, I come without any feeling."

"I lack the spirit to live."

"I always go by what is expected of me. At the same time, I keep everything away from myself, while at the same time losing myself."

Later in therapy, she says: "I keep noticing that I protect myself by not expecting anything from others at all. I have to make do myself."

Still later, she says: "I notice how I instinctively resist being moved by what you say. I notice how I want to reject you." (She appropriately gestures with her hands.)

I sense:

The patient makes it to my office, but the moment we meet confronts her with something she cannot fulfill. She is fundamentally overwhelmed. How is she supposed to face me if she has no inner space where I can await her entry, where I can already anticipate her coming? If she arrives as someone "without any feeling" (see above), she necessarily finds herself in a space without any emotional horizon, without any expectations. How does that work? Well, it doesn't work at all – except for the banal emergency stop to the whole affair, squeezed into the template: "Now it's greeting time." The patient tries to belie the emptiness by pretending something that does not exist: a familiarity through a buddy-like closeness. She attempts to cope with the situation with such a leap of faith. But, basically, she is completely helpless and destitute. Since she lacks a responsive self that can define itself in the relationship, she lacks the means to carefully examine whether she can take me up on my offer in the form of responding (cf. Waldenfels, 2016 [2007], pp. 477, 505, 614). She is exposed to the events quite abruptly, without a filter, head-on, without any protection. Thus, if she is to "survive," all that remains is to frigidly advance wearing her clinging-rejecting armor without wavering or fine-tuning. She uses all of this to escape an affect lurking in the background: crushing shame. After all, she clearly feels that something is not working – that's why she sought therapy. But no matter how hard she tries, her therapist and everyone else in her immediate surroundings live in a different world, supported by conventions that do not exist for her. What impertinence: a space of potential relationships to which she has no access.

Giving Space to What Does Not Work

It took me a long time to completely understand what was being expressed, for example, in the patient's tardiness. It lay, well hidden in open sight, projecting no more and no less than: "Things can't start between us as they do with the others." I had to understand that this truth manifested itself in the antagonistic action of always being late. It referred to the absence of something natural, something the patient feared – perhaps rightly so – would be ignored and betrayed if she were to simply arrive on time and without a fuss at her "session with me" (cf. Küchenhoff, 2012, pp. 317ff.). Of course, this would mean the patient, who could not imagine my waiting for her arrival, would still ensure that I was, in fact, already waiting because of her habitual lateness. Anything else would have precipitated a catastrophe. In the end, these realizations on my part had something liberating about them. So, it wasn't classic resistance. It calmed me and lifted the pressure of expectation that I, now frustrated, had probably presented to the patient more often than she could tolerate. I had to understand that I had hung the interpretive pattern of projective identification – the tension I felt while waiting for someone who was not (yet) there, including anger, rage, and frustration – a little too high and assumed an "agent" who did not yet exist in this way (cf. Press, 2021, p. 119). Nevertheless, it turned out to be a lengthy process. More often than I would have liked, I struggled at feeling devalued or dominated, impatiently wondering what was being delayed *again*, what was holding her back *again*, what she was trying to deflect …

Little by little, I had to learn to deal with the circumstance that, at the beginning of each session, we entered a situation in which we were physically in the same room but without actually responding to each other yet. My greatest difficulty was perceiving and accepting the situation as it truly was. I wanted the patient to be *different* (cf. Bion, 1970, p. 56), and precisely this wish exposed me even more to a state of powerlessness, helplessness, and probably also unintentionally friendly intrusiveness on my part, against which the patient felt compelled to defend herself.

Room for Development

The fact that, in good moments, there existed a basis between the patient and me that fundamentally enables a space for "things that don't work" made careful development possible in the back-and-forth of small steps. Even at the beginning of therapy, this sometimes occurred within a single session. Out of a paralyzed, stagnant relationship that kept us stuck in the same old same, there developed, albeit haltingly, a means of devoting time to something that was not yet there. This allowed something to form that gradually made the therapy room feel more like a waiting room for the soul, where nothing was happening (yet) but perhaps *could* happen. Later, there emerged the friendly image of a mother holding her child by the hand who stood on the precipice of things and needed some time to grasp what was to come. So, I just breathe and wait with her. Being alienated was now not associated with being lost, but rather was enveloped by a vague feeling of concomitant closeness. This eventually led to the patient and me observing our situation in unison and coming to an understanding about the "not yet."

During one session, the patient is talking about something but suddenly stops to say that she has just realized she is not really there yet. Another time she greets me with a smile, then falls back into rigidity, but remarks, "I don't know if I'm there yet, I don't think I'm there yet." In all of these scenes, as paradoxical as it may sound, she has already related to me as the one who is not yet there. At the same time, the patient is freed from the effort of having to be someone to me who conforms to expectations. On the contrary, together we can experience and understand how the patient succeeds in remaining true to herself because "it is not yet possible" and not overplay anything in these moments. In another session, in turn, her fixed gaze relaxes, and I hear her say, "I have to look at you first." Her path to me now takes on a temporal dimension that yields the possibility of actually arriving at me. This is matched by her gaze taking on a searching, groping quality in this tender moment; the frosty caginess disappears – and now my gaze can meet hers inquiringly. During such passages, the temperature between us changes – it becomes warmer. Yet, if I then try to approach her, I experience her gaze immediately closing me out, accompanied by a dismissive hand gesture. Again, I'm back on my own, having entertained illusions, wanting too much too quickly, and having to deal with my disappointment. In the shrinking process of perceived rejection, I try to remain true to my body by attending to my breathing without withdrawing from the patient. But that is not easy: I, too, am vulnerable in my answer-seeking motions (cf. Waldenfels, 2002, pp. 117ff.). In the end, we engage through the patient's ability to put these events between us as well into words: "I notice how I instinctively resist being touched by what you say. I notice how I want to reject you."

Fathoming

Toward the end of therapy, during several sessions, the patient looks at me deeply. The word that comes to mind today for this situation is fathoming. By this, I do not mean a cognitive effort or her wanting to know something, but rather her search for depth, for somewhere to anchor herself to, in the true sense of fathoming, in the depths of intercorporeity. The situation demands that I let myself be fathomed. Her gaze does not mean she is seeking to comprehend the therapist Jörg Scharff as the patient believes to already know him within the framework of the therapeutic setting. Rather, her gaze seeks to fathom me directly. It is one of intimacy and simultaneously one of exposed innocence that gives me no place to hide or withdraw. I have no choice (cf. Stern, 2005, p. 175). This timeless, craving gaze is open to something that is to be given substantially by me. I struggle with a fear of failure: What if this becomes too intense or goes on too long – can I even live up to it? And if I do approach her, who from my past am I looking to find? Inner objects intertwine, I become anxious. How far can I go and still be myself? Is this even permissible? For the duration of these moments, her gaze queries me about our capacity for love – hers and mine – and she surrenders to this question. But this cannot go on for very long, since eroticism inevitably sprouts up. Despite all the probing, in the end something unfathomable remains: a feeling of "near you and yet so far," a kind of distant closeness (cf. Waldenfels, 2002, p. 86). And precisely this turn of events makes me feel that, despite all the surrendering, something is also withdrawing, withholding itself, which brings us back to our separateness. Then relief ensues that it is possible to return from this borderline situation. I find myself in with her for moments that transcend the usual therapeutic asymmetry of the given framework. Overall, it is healing. In a later session, the patient says, "Something has emerged that cannot be willed."

In those moments, when the relationship evolved into the "primary relationship" (Kinston & Cohen, 1987, pp. 34ff.), because of the extensive absence of any defense, the patient not infrequently felt herself completely at the mercy of an unexpected intrusion. During one session, I formulated her problems in an external relationship – which was accompanied by violent ambivalent tendencies while her newly won love relationship with the world sought its place – once again to the effect that, if she expected nothing, she would indeed be completely at the mercy of current events. At that moment, my patient felt deeply touched by what I had said – and, quite unexpectedly, precisely what I had spoken about happened. She struggles for words and says I had voiced and understood something important, for which she is very grateful to me. At the same time, she begins to cry, flooded with blushes of shame. It seems as if, in the moment of feeling understood, being touched and being flooded cannot be separated from each other. Her inner world of imaginative anticipation, which would allow a gradual appropriation and representation of the event, is only in the process of being established (cf. Waldenfels, 2002, pp. 323ff.). The patient feels naked and bare the blood-red heat in her cheeks probably both expresses archaic shame and serves as a saving grace. So, how do I look at this moment? I lower my gaze. I wait. Inwardly, I wrap the patient in a blanket that contains the fire and later try to look at her with a warm gaze. Was I successful?

At the beginning of a session, the patient takes a deep breath: This is a test of her resolve. I hold my breath – what will she confide in me? Hesitantly, she notes that, in the previous hour, I had closed my eyes for a while. This had irritated her. She had the feeling that I was blocking her out. Relieved, I return that I am glad she is telling me about her irritation. Therein lies a sign of trust: She is building a bridge to me. For my part, I can totally understand her insecurity; eyes are indeed something like doors through which we enter and leave. At the same time, however, closing my eyes helped me to reflect differently, and in a certain way, I felt even closer to her. Inwardly, I keep looking at her: Does that help her to surrender herself to such a moment? She understands what I am trying to say, but it is different with her: She *needs* my gaze, she says emphatically.

Again, the difficulty of internally representing the attention of the other remains in the background. The crisis experienced by the patient at such moments is by no means trivial. She feels supported by my gaze, so if I close my eyes, our relationship no longer exists, and she feels blanked out. This should not be understood metaphorically: The patient experiences my physically closing my eyes, as a concrete act in which I "disappear her" from the world. What is new, however, is that the abyss she falls into does not remain unuttered. Rather, the patient confesses her various feelings to me and fights emphatically to preserve the relationship: "I *need* your gaze!" Could this admission mark the beginning of a development, where one day she no longer needs my gaze in this way?

In the next session, she returns to this passage in another context and again recapitulates that she had addressed me because of my gaze. I said to her, "You were calling me to you." The patient is deeply moved, and tears come to her eyes. "That I even said that … " The patient is so touched by my words that it overwhelms her again. How is she supposed to take precautions against something happening to her immediately (cf. Waldenfels, 2002, p. 62)? Then she catches herself and says, "I myself would never have said it like that, or maybe just a little bit." In her postscript – "or maybe just a little bit" – she once again expresses her own concern.

Sometime later, in anticipation of a summary comment, when I conclude by remarking that maybe this is again a little too much, she surprises me with a spontaneous reply something like: No, she would like me to tackle a topic; in fact, she would like me to "tackle" her; she also experiences this elsewhere. She has come to notice how receptive she is to it, even needs it. She looks at me with an attentive curiosity full of liveliness. In such situations, she feels the back-and-forth that arises in her – she emphasizes the last sentence with a corresponding hand movement.

Thus, the patient and I retain in grateful remembrance what can be possible in a therapeutic relationship.

Note

1   See, among others, Goetzmann and Ruettner (2007), pp. 138ff.; Leikert (2019), p. 127; Lemma (2018), pp. 191ff.; Press (2021), pp. 118 f.; Scharff (2010), pp. 189 f.; Scharff (2021), pp. 19ff.; Schultz-Venrath (2021), p. 189; Volz-Boers (2016), pp. 141 f.

References

Bion, W. R. (1970): *Attention and Interpretation*. London: Tavistock. German.
Goetzmann, L. & Ruettner, B. (2007): Explosionen, Beton, Totes und "Schrumpfungsprozesse" – zur Focusing-Wahrnehmung des Körpers in der Gegenübertragung. *Psyche – Z Psychoanal*, 61(2), 137–150.
Kinston, W. & Cohen, J. (1987): *Urverdrängung und andere seelische Zustände. Der Bereich der Psychostatik*. Vortrag auf der Arbeitstagung der deutschen psychoanalytischen Vereinigung, Wiesbaden, 19–21 November 1987.
Küchenhoff, J. (2012): *Körper und Sprache. Theoretische und klinische Beiträge zu einem intersubjektiven Verständnis des Körpererlebens*. Gießen: Psychosozial.
Leikert, S. (2019): *Das sinnliche Selbst. Das Körpergedächtnis in der psychoanalytischen Behandlungstechnik*. Frankfurt a. M.: Brandes & Apsel.
Lemma, A. (2018): *Der Körper spricht immer. Körperlichkeit in psychoanalytischen Therapien und jenseits der Couch*. Trans. by L. Apsel. Frankfurt a. M.: Brandes & Apsel.
Press, J. (2021): Der analytische Prozess zwischen Öffnung zum Formlosen und Suche nach Sinn. *Psyche – Z Psychoanal*, 75, 105–131.
Scharff, J. M. (2010): *Die leibliche Dimension in der Psychoanalyse*. Frankfurt a. M.: Brandes & Apsel.
Scharff, J. M. (2021): *Psychoanalyse und Zwischenleiblichkeit. Klinisch-propädeutisches Seminar*. Frankfurt a. M.: Brandes & Apsel.
Schneider, G. (2006): Ein "'unmöglicher' Beruf" (Freud) – zur aporetischen Grundlegung der psychoanalytischen Behandlungstechnik und ihrer Entwicklung. *Psyche – Z Psychoanal*, 60, 900–931.
Schultz-Venrath, U. (2021): *Mentalisieren des Körpers*. Stuttgart: Klett-Cotta.
Staehle, A. (2009): "In Schweigen oder Worte hülle ich mich ein." Von autistischen Barrieren zu Worten mit Bedeutung oder von der Ungetrenntheit zur Differenzierung zwischen Selbst und Anderen. In: Nissen, B. (Ed.): *Die Entstehung des Psychischen. Psychoanalytische Perspektiven*. Gießen: Psychosozial, 167–192.
Stern, D. N. (2005): *Der Gegenwartsmoment. Veränderungsprozesse in Psychoanalyse, Psychotherapie und Alltag*. Trans. by E. Vorspohl. Frankfurt a. M.: Brandes & Apsel. 5th ed. 2018.
Volz-Boers, U. (2016): Resonanz im Körper des Analytikers. Das Konzept der sensorisch intuitiven Haltung. In: Walz-Pawlita, S., Unruh, B. & Janta, B. (Eds.): *Körper-Sprachen*. Gießen: Psychosozial, 141–152.
Waldenfels, B. (2002): *Bruchlinien der Erfahrung*. Frankfurt a. M.: Suhrkamp.
Waldenfels, B. (2016 [2007]): *Antwortregister*. Frankfurt a. M.: Suhrkamp.

Chapter 5

Accidents of Seduction and the Theory of the Body

Christophe Dejours

In this contribution, I would like to talk about the body from two points of view:

- as a target of certain psychopathological decompensations and
- as a metapsychological concept.

I begin with a clinical fragment concerning an acute somatic decompensation in a patient who has been in analysis for 5 years, his second installment after an initial 7-year analysis with me. Between the two analyses, there was a 7-year gap. Both were classical analyses, with three sessions per week on the couch. From an analysis of the symptom, I proceed to explore the theoretical questions raised by the metapsychological status of the body, including a discussion of the genealogy of the erotic body. I attempt to identify what might be called "accidents of seduction" in the communication between the child and the adult, hindering the emergence of the erotic body. These are accidents that arguably then shape the body through an elective vulnerability to targeted somatic decompensation; a vulnerability whose identification in the course of analysis might point toward a path capable of restarting the formation of the erotic body.

A Clinical Fragment

Maurice Garance has missed several analysis sessions. He had just experienced an acute episode of vertigo that required hospitalization for several days in the neurology department – which occurs precisely on Saint Maurice Day. He had taken advantage of the offer of an "open day" at an organic farm, and after enjoying a hearty lunch on the estate, he went outdoors under a blazing sun. Then, after lunch, he drives his car to facilities at the other end of the estate, drops his wife off at the meeting place, and drives off again to park his car in the nearby parking lot.

Suddenly, he is seized with a feeling of imminent death, accompanied by extreme dizziness, nausea, severe abdominal pain, and vomiting. Despite the

DOI: 10.4324/9781003370130-5

strong physical discomfort and the feeling that his demise is imminent, the thought occurs to him to press the horn of his vehicle to try to summon someone. An elderly man approaches, and Mr. Garance asks him to call his wife, giving him her first name. A few minutes later, she appears, and he asks her to take him to the emergency room of the nearest hospital. The ride there goes badly. They must stop because he starts having convulsions, during which he loses all control, vomiting and defecating. But the situation only worsens, so they stop the car and contact emergency services, which send an ambulance to pick him up.

The electrocardiogram at the hospital is normal. An emergency CT scan is ordered, but it, too, is unremarkable. The neurological examination reveals marked nystagmus, and he remains hospitalized on the neurology ward. After 3 days of further examinations and observation, during which he constantly feels suspended between life and death, the doctors produce a diagnosis of peripheral neurological disorder: acute vestibular neuritis of unknown, probably viral, origin, which they expect to recede.

In the first analysis session, after a break of several weeks, his associations produce a detailed account of the circumstances of the somatic crisis. He had been sitting at a large table in the sun; it was very hot that day. Perhaps sunstroke?

Then he is reminded of his fear of death and describes in detail, especially how he thought he was experiencing his own death. Thereupon, he had to go through all the steps of returning to Earth or experiencing a new birth. He had to learn to eat again, beginning with liquids, then learn to walk again, tottering like a child, without little sense of balance, etc. Then he gets angry about Saint Mauritius Day, recalling that he had once had somatic problems on that day several years ago. He recounts the story of the first name of his paternal grandfather, which was given to him so that said grandfather, who had died long ago, would not be forgotten, etc. For several days now, he said, he has had intense dreams, night after night.

He interrupts his story to recount a circumstantial detail and begins to talk about his eyes. In the hospital, he had to stay in bed the whole time and keep his eyes closed for several days. When he opened his eyes once again, he became extremely dizzy. Even now, he says, he still suffers from severe eye fatigue. He thinks this is because his eyes have witnessed the whole cycle of death, life, and rebirth ... He feels that, by resting and regaining his eyesight, he might be able to recover.

And then, as he continues to associate, the following question comes to mind: He wonders if his camera might not have caused this accident. He had taken many photos that day and had felt that something like an electric current had emanated from the camera, which could have triggered the neurological problems. Afterward, he took his camera to a photographer to have it examined, by the way.

At that point, I lose my cool a little bit. After all, we are dealing with nothing more than a *delusion*. In combination with a somatic decompensation!

I decide to intervene, saying that this whole history of Saint Mauritius and its anniversary does not seem to me to be essential. On the other hand, the thing with the camera seems much more worrisome. For a long time, we have known (more or less vaguely) that his predilection for photography is related to his sexual interests; the sadistic exhibitionism of his father, who indulged in downright butchery in front of his son, plays a role here. In the past, he had frequently photographed his girlfriend naked in lewd postures and positions. It should be emphasized, however, that this new knack for photography came to light only during the analysis.

My comments astonish him extraordinarily. Nevertheless, he begins to speak once again: At the beginning of the summer, he says, he went on a trip alone. He visited a female friend who lives in the province. She told him about all her difficulties in life, especially her very troublesome vascular problems. She bleeds very quickly. She used to suffer from DIC (disseminated intravascular coagulopathy), one after effect of which is that sexual intercourse triggers vaginal bleeding. "No one can touch me," she told him. This sentence struck and impressed him very much. No one can touch her – and yet she had prepared for Mr. Garance to sleep in her bed. During his stay with her, she effectively forced him to sleep in her bed, while she herself slept on the sofa. He didn't want this arrangement, but she insisted. And during the day, when she went to work, he traveled around the area. He went to a nearby town to see the exhibition of plasticized corpses.[1]

During a meal on the farm, about a week after the visit to visit his bleeding friend, he found himself sitting at the table with a couple, and the woman was red-headed. And very beautiful! He took lots of pictures of her. So, he especially likes redheads? (This detail was unknown to me until then.) His answer is not long in coming: His female friend from the province is also a redhead – and fantastically beautiful to boot.

He had the pictures developed. But because of the flash, everybody has red pupils!

Strangely enough, when he was in the house of the bleeding friend, in this strange state of mind – lots of red hair, beauty, desire, and forbidden touching – he developed a kind of fever blister in his mouth, likely lip herpes.

So, in the end, we have a parallel concatenation: The first is the *traumatic* time spent with his female friend in the province, the redheadedness, the beauty, the intimacy, the blood, the bleeding, and the "do not touch" edict (The right only to contemplate). Then herpes sets in. A week later, he meets up with a new redhead, new beauty, new closeness, new prohibition of touching, and all blood-red pupils in all the photos. So, in *duplicity and after the fact*, a neurological crisis is triggered (probably against the background of a developing virosis that came to a head).

There's a message somewhere in this encounter, but this message is not translatable. Why? Because it reaches Mr. Garance during a time of "proscription" (I return to this term later), the zone where blood-precipitating violence is intensified by being mixed with exsanguination, sadism, death, and no doubt murder and sexual desire. Based on what I know about this patient, I cannot help but associate this message with the father's enigmatic behavior with the violent, sadistic, murderous, and destructive acts he perpetrated on the bodies of his animal victims. Something about the two redheaded women points to the untranslatable message of their habitus (to the "accidental seduction") and to the mental paralysis the patient experienced as a child when confronted with his father's seduction, formulated through an action that reveals the desire for death, murder, and blood-letting.

The father was a serious hunter who incessantly killed game, whereupon the son would have to come, fill a bowl with wine, and hold it while he *plucked out the eye of a rabbit*, grabbed it by its hind legs, and let the blood drip directly into the bowl. (Remember the redheaded woman's red eyes and Mr. Garance's voyeurism.)

The other screen memory is the day the father called the son into the garage and had him set up two benches, on which he laid the dog with the *reddish-brown* fur and shot it in the head in front of his son.

The Standard Theory

This clinical fragment raises the question of the relationships between a somatic crisis, a psychotic crisis, and sexuality. Conventional psychosomatic theory is unable to take into account the complexity of the phenomena at play here. This patient, Mr. Garance, does not function mentally "opératoire" (i.e., mechanistically) (Marty & de M'Uzan, 1963). His decompensation does not occur in the context of an essential depression; indeed, it is far from it (Marty, 1968). We could investigate the causes in terms of economic mutations and reorganizations, but from a clinical point of view, that approach fails to emphasize the economic dimension in any way and does not seem wise. True, taking an economic view or even explicitly relying on an economic vantage point is sometimes necessary when interpreting a situation or a clinical configuration. But that is particularly valid when the patient's associations have already been exhausted at the beginning of the session – when the patient sticks to strictly describing the medical and surgical events, avoiding other associations and cursory ideas: When the patient does not want to search and is not driven by curiosity toward his own functioning. In other words, when the patient refuses to offer the analyst any space for interpretations, he spontaneously displays no astonishment at the affective and psychic dimensions of his own behavior. Analysts trained in the standard theory of psychosomatics then shift their attention to the economic aspects available to psychoanalytic listening, which consequently tends to degenerate into observing economic semiology, something Michel Fain and Pierre Marty were very fond of (Marty et al., 1968): A semiology that, in some respects, resembles more a medical view of signs than a psychoanalytic perspective (in the strict sense). In short, analytic listening cedes its place to semiological expertise.

In contrast, the clinical fragment of severe somatic decompensation presented above is part of a lively conjuncture of association in which the self-preservation instinct – which Freud says is subordinate to the interests of the ego – has not collapsed. Mr. Garance, feeling impending death in the middle of a crisis, frantically honked the horn of his car to summon help. And he succeeded!

An Analysis of the Conflict and the Hypothesis of the "Constitutional Factor"

So, let's leave the economic path and take another perspective, pursuing first of all the classical means of interpreting the conflict. This orientation is justified and indeed warranted because of the critical episode that brings the patient's actual sexual issues to the fore. But in the case at hand, Mr. Garance's crisis does not manifest itself in the form of impotence; we are not dealing here with a simple vasovagal malaise. There is no hysterical conversion. And yet, the course of the drive movements is remarkably similar in many respects: Instead of a conversion, we observe a labyrinth of neuritis and the beginning of a processual psychotic episode. So, at first glance, everything looks like we are dealing with hysteria "with a bad outcome" – with a failed conversion.

But why this drift into somatic illness and delusion? The most tempting, because the simplest, explanation would be that the psychopathological movement in question is indeed based on hysteria, but that the tendency toward the somatic-psychotic stems from the "breeding ground," from the idiosyncrasy, the constitutional factor, as Freud would have said: from the "somatic accommodation" – a term as enigmatic as they come.

This version certainly has some truth, but this reading may also be wrong. By attributing the inference to somatose psychosis to the constitutional factor, we are de facto conceding that we are in the realm of the unanalyzable, i.e., that the problem of the relationship(s) between neurosis, psychosis, somatosis, and sexuality lies entirely beyond the reach of psychoanalysis. That would amount to taking another step backward, behind standard psychosomatics, which at least has the merit of suggesting there is a path leading out of the impasse of the unanalyzable: by employing the economic aspect in psychosomatics or even in psychoanalysis in general.

Refusing to take up the explanation by the constitutional factor would mean opening the black box of the constitution. Is this constitution "constitutional"? That would be the biologizing explanation. If this constitution were the result of a "transmission of innateness," it would be the phylogenetic explanation Freud prefers in order to introduce the famous primordial fantasies. The constitutional factor would act as a vestige of the transgenerational transmission of a conflictual etiology reaching back to the origins, if not of humankind, then at least of a lineage, of a family: to a kind of evil spell that, as we would say for the House of Areus, trickles down to the descendants starting from the history of the founder of the lineage.

Many analysts subscribe to this hypothesis, some openly by speaking of familial archetypes, whereas others resort (more or less precisely) to a notion of transgenerational transmission from unconscious to unconscious. The most sophisticated of these versions stems from Torok and Abraham (Torock, 1978) with their "phantoms thesis."

I can present little scientific argumentation to refute the constitutional factor thesis, which provides a kind of "all-purpose" explanation that can be invoked when all other interpretations have reached an impasse. Yet, it has the disadvantage of not being open to criticism. In short, my dislike stems largely from the fact that I do not share this conviction.

From "Constitution" to the Genealogy of the Erogenous Body

A problem then pops up in an entirely different form: What is the origin of this constitutional factor, viz., in Mr. Garance's history (and not in that of his ancestors)? Or also: How did this constitution emerge (in Mr. Garance's childhood)? To answer this question, I propose a theory that incorporates something I have already alluded to in the title of this contribution, the "accidents of seduction." Such accidents would be nothing more than accidents that occur during the formation of the sexual unconscious, well known from the framework of Jean Laplanche's (1997) general theory of seduction.

All told, it represents a way of accounting for how the basic anthropological situation, which assigns to the adult the position of seducer and to the child that of interpreter, cripples the child's ability to translate those messages compromised by the adult's sexual unconscious.

In 1990, Jean Laplanche wrote a short text on this subject matter (2017a [1992]) using the term "intromission" to describe this process, as opposed to the usual process described by the "implantation" of the message.

What is the implantation of a message? In general seduction theory, the basis of communication between the child and the adult is structured by a particular drive much discussed in contemporary literature, namely, that of attachment. Attachment is an innate behavioral constellation that leads the child toward the adult's body, strictly in the sense of the self-preservation instinct. Seen from this perspective, the self-preservation instinct is not solipsistic but communicative from the outset. To the appeal emanating from the child's body, which seeks skin contact, warmth, and an energetic substrate, the adult responds with nurture (today we would say "care"). The ethological basis of this behavior is what Bowlby describes with the term "retrieval."

Nevertheless, the adult who cares for the child's body does not react to it on a purely hygienic-nutritional level. The adult cannot persist on the strictly instrumental level of body care because every adult has a sexual unconscious. The reaction of the adult to the body of the summoning child is therefore initially certainly instrumental. And, on the level of self-preservation, this constitutes the adult's message to the child in response to the child's appeal, which is carried by the attachment "wave." But this response message is *compromised* by the adult's sexual unconscious. As a result, the adult's message is contaminated with sexuality and, nolens volens, assumes the form of a message compromised by unconscious sexuality. That is the "compromised message," also called the "enigmatic message."

When adults enter into this body-to-body situation with a child, which takes place at the level of "grooming," the adults arouse the child's body with their sometimes supple, sometimes stiff, sometimes caressing gestures, with the music of their voice, and with their smells. The adult's entire body is involved, including their – the adult's – sexuality.

This very moment of body-to-body interaction is the moment when the adult's message is *implanted* in the child. Such implantation presents the compromised message with a sensual dimension, the subtext to the message, giving it the status of an enigmatic message.

The child does all the rest: The translation of the message! In this second round of translation, the child translates as much as possible and as completely as possible, but there always remains an untranslated remainder, a translation shadow, which is deposited in the child and constitutes the child's sexual unconscious: the translational theory of the unconscious and the translational theory of primal repression.[2] I would like to emphasize that, from this perspective, the repressed sexual unconscious of the child, stemming from the child's ability/inability to correctly translate the message, depends quite fundamentally on the child's own mind. According to this conception, there is no direct transference from the adult's unconscious to that of the child, and there is no transgenerational reproduction whatsoever. Interposed between the adult and the child is always the child's own mind, that is, the child's mode of translation. What becomes of the compromised message transmitted by the adult's unconscious is completely unpredictable. Ultimately, everything depends on how the child translates it. So, there is no passing on from one generation to another, no ancestral curse. (A rose sometimes grows from a dunghill.)

The path I just evoked is the *usual* fate of the message: via implantation to the emergence of the *repressed sexual unconscious*.

The Concept of the "Intromission" of the Message in the General Theory of Seduction

In response to objections long addressed to him, Laplanche briefly mentions situations in which translation completely fails – radical untranslatability – which, in a sense, reflect the exception to the rule, the exception to the general theory of seduction. Instead of implantation, in this context, he speaks of "intromission," which *leaves in the child something to be translated*, something that has remained wholly untranslated and lies at the origin of the nonneurotic pathologies.

Agreed!

I propose to expand on this theme and emphasize the radical untranslated as an accident of the child's seduction by the adult. In this perspective, the child must translate not the compromised message of the adult but the *effect* that compromised message has on the child's body. In other words, the child primarily translates the bodily states emerging from the adult's state of arousal. Hence, the formulas: "Thinking originally always means thinking one's own body" and "thinking the bodily experience I have." The prototype of such a thought connection would precisely be translating my very own bodily experience that will never be anything other than my own. An experience that is not observable from without is not objectifiable, is not visible, and will always remain so, as part of the absolute subjectivity of life that experiences itself: in the mode of a *pâtir* (suffering), a passion, a radical passivity that is primary, primordial, and precedes all thought, all *cogito*.

Yet, what must be mobilized is what is presented to the ego (or for the ego), which constitutes itself through this very act of translation, between the primary experience of the body, which experiences itself in the darkness of subjective nonseeing, on the one hand, and its translation, on the other hand. What is called for is no more and no less than a psychic work in the strict sense, also an act of *binding* excitement: Excitement that manifests itself in the body precisely in the form of sensual pleasure. As Freud writes, there is room here for a measure of the "work demand" imposed on the psychic apparatus by virtue of its connection with the body (Freud, 1915c). The formation of the drive goes hand in hand with that of the self. At the same time, repression through translation forms, on the one hand, the unconscious and, on the other hand, the preconscious – the self.

As the wielder of a primary power of translation, the body intervenes at this point. Indeed, it is the body that receives the message by implementation; it is the body that feels the sensual excitation; and it is the body that carries the ability to initialize a translation, something Freud only vaguely sensed when he wrote that the ego is originally a superficial entity, a body-self:

> The ego is ultimately derived from bodily sensations, chiefly from those springing from the surface of the body. It may thus be regarded as a mental projection of the surface of the body, besides, as we have seen above, representing the superficies of the mental apparatus." In the English edition of *The Ego and the Id* of 1927, Freud added this note to the original text, which read: " The ego is first and foremost a bodily ego; it is not merely a surface entity, but is itself the projection of a surface. (Freud, 1923b, p. 26)

My impression is that Freud only had an inkling of the problem but did not develop it any further. Anzieu (1985) gave it its most complete form with his theory of the "skin-ego." For my part, I would look in a somewhat different direction than Anzieu, namely, employing the theory of the "thinking body" from the philosophy of principles, based on the simple act of "perceptible effort" and brilliantly developed by Maine de Biran from the concept of "immediate apperception" over 200 years ago.

Unfortunately, I cannot discuss this point in greater depth here but would like to point out the general direction for further theoretical investigation (de Biran, 1995 [1807]).

The Notion of the Libidinal Subversion of the Physiological Body

Returning to metapsychology, let us imagine a theory of the formation of the erotic body that starts from the other "simple fact" described by Freud (1905d) in terms of the anaclisis of drive on/to the physiological function. This is a subtle process: A child tries to show their parents that, for example, their mouth is an organ that serves not only the function of consuming food, but it also serves the child for sucking, kissing, biting, and later the little games of sexual life. Thus, the subject affirms a certain independence of this organ – the mouth – from its original purpose, using it not only when hungry but sometimes also when seeking pleasure. At the same time, the subject discovers that they are not a slave to their instincts and needs, not just an animal organism, but that they can become the subject of desire. One can see that the anaclitic functions as a subversion: The mouth, the fulcrum of subversion, comes to be recognized as an erogenous zone. Of course, we are dealing with an *organ* here and not a *function*. To be more or less liberated from the dictatorship of a physiological function, we need the organ as a necessary mediator: *The subversion of the function by the drive takes place by way of the organ.*

Freud described the successive phases[3] in the development of sexuality. Step by step, in this process, various parts of the body offer themselves for anaclasis and prove to be erogenous zones. Gradually, these zones are snatched from their natural masters – their physiological functions – to be subverted and construct what is called the subjective or *erotic body*. For this process, I propose the term "libidinous subversion," which denotes the subversion of the physiological role in favor of the erotic role. Via just such a development of psychological sexuality, the subject manages to partially free itself from its physiological functions, automatic behaviors, and even its biological rhythms: To a certain extent, at least, human sexuality manages to override endocrinal and metabolic rhythms. In women, for example, sexuality no longer follows the menstrual cycle, nor does it end with menopause. Libidinous subversion allows the register of desire to establish primacy over the need.

However, we must note that the subversive conquest of the physiological by the erotic body always remains unfinished business. Mental sexuality and erotic economy often risk becoming "misaligned," detaching themselves from the alignment and generating a counterrevolutionary act that causes the serious decompensations that force us to reflect on a theory of the body in psychoanalysis.

Not to forget the essential influence of the relationships the child establishes with the adult. From this perspective, the development of the erotic body results from a dialog concerning the body and its functions based on the bodily care the child receives from the adult.

Here is where *the genealogy of the subjective body* becomes clear. The whole process unfolds within the relationship with the other. However, psychoanalysis suggests that this relationship is innately *unequal* (Ferenczi, 2004 [1932]; Laplanche, 2011 [1987]). And the main interface between the child and the adult is the body: body care and body games.

Even if the instrumental theme regarding exchanges between the adult and the child in the objective world lies primarily in the quality of care, through its very nature, this relationship inevitably brings about the emergence of other aspects: pleasure, desire, arousal, and, in a broader sense, the entire erotic dimension, which cannot be seen separately from the body games. The second body, the erotic one, emerges from the first one, the physiological body. Between the two lies all the handling and gesturing of the adult regarding the child's body.

Accidents of Seduction

In this scenario – a prototranslation at the body level through body games between the child and the adult as a means of early mental appropriation by the ego of something experienced affectively in the body – accidental seduction occurs when the adult is flooded by the excitement the child's body arouses in them.

That is to say, when the adult gets carried away by an uncontrollable, unbridled, and unconscious reaction in the face of the appeal of the child's body, the child can no longer translate the message. For example, when the adult suddenly feels an uncontrollable aversion reaction toward the child's body, leading them to hit the child; or when, in order to avoid that happening, the adult suddenly and icily retreats and breaks off communication; or, when overly aroused by the child, the adult gets carried away and sexually abuses the child's body. This is the specific situation Laplanche had in mind when he chose to conceptualize intromission during his 2006 lecture in Vienna (Laplanche, 2017d).

The Two Types of Unconscious

What are the consequences of an adult's violence against a child's body, regarding the topological aspect? First of all, the message remains untranslated, though that may not even be the most important thing. The experience the body has here inscribes itself in the body as an excess of excitement leading to destabilization of or even a rupture of the ego – an ego, being still in the process of formation. The event inscribes itself exclusively in the body, as something that, by its very nature, lodges in a functional register that is dangerous and threatening to the psychic integrity of the ego. Summa summarum, an uninhabitable island, develops in the body – in the form of impossible body games. I call this process *proscription* to indicate the fundamental difference from *repression*. The latter is translational and takes the route via the child's *pensée* (which subsumes thinking and mental/psychological processing), leading, at the topical level, to a differentiation between the repressed sexual unconscious and the preconscious. Proscription, on the other hand, stands outside any possible means of translational processing and contributes to the formation of impossible registers of bodily functioning, of zones of paresis, paralysis, and death, or of danger to life in the aforementioned body games. In adult sexuality, these zones become translated into the registers, striking the subject with frigidity and making them feel the sense of death at every touch, a sense of life departing, of a cold body on withdrawal. This cruel experience is one of a deep chasm, like that of the figure in Hesiod's *Theogonies*: The fear of falling endlessly (Dejours, 2004), which at times can escalate to mental confusion (amentia) or delusion, but more often to a bout of somatic illness.

If translation is impossible because of the overexcitement that has precipitated a crisis situation for the child in the first place, what is inscribed in the body's experience does not subsequently lead to a translation and thus also not to the formation of a repressed sexual unconscious. What happens here completely eludes repression and, by extension, the realm of the psychosexual. Rather, it causes another form of the unconscious to be formed, which I propose designating as the "amential" unconscious.

In the case of Mr. Garance, this analysis allows us to return to the moment when that nucleus of the amential unconscious formed, to the moment when the somatic and psychotic reactions presented in this one episode first appeared.

To the appeal of the little boy Mr. Garance once was, his father, carried away by a wild homosexual reaction, finds no other reaction than to terrify his son by inviting him to witness bloody slaughter scenes that frighten and paralyze the child such that he loses all self-control and soils himself. Whereupon the father threatens him further with violent acts he inflicts on the bodies of the animals.

Such accidents of communication between the child and the adult sometimes occur very early in life. Yet clinical experience suggests that, although they can devastatingly affect the formation of the erotic body in ways that last late into life, they are especially damaging during puberty, when the adult goes crazy in light of the adolescent body.

One of the essential characteristics of such excesses of excitement that come crashing down on the child is that they carry a formidable threat: The danger of decompensation of the adult, perhaps triggered by the child's body games. The fragility zone of the child's body, which on a topical level corresponds to the amential unconscious, is simultaneously a zone that bears the stamp of the threat of physical violence in the form of rape or infanticide.

Working Through the Amential Unconscious

To bring this account to an end (albeit not a conclusion, for I cannot list all the intermediate links here), the amential unconscious may not lie entirely beyond the reach of analytic reworking after all. I am convinced that the scission between the sector formed by the repressed unconscious and the preconscious, on the one hand, and the sector occupied by the amential unconscious, on the other hand, is present in every human being. Sometimes, this scission lasts a lifetime; sometimes, it becomes destabilized, as evidenced by episodes of decompensation such as that of Mr. Garance. If analysis is properly continued, part of what lurks in the amential unconscious can be repatriated from one sector to the other, thus becoming available to translation, which in turn allows recapturing those body games previously "*proscribed.*" The most important thing in this process is not for the analyst to someday provide the patient with an exhaustive interpretation, but that the patients themselves do a very specific form of mental work. This work takes place through dreamwork, by "working through the dream," the character-istics of which can be specified.

Sometime after the delirious and somatic incident described, Mr. Garance reports a dream after experiencing pain in his thigh during the session, which he attributes to tendonitis from walking too much in the days before. He continually thinks about this pain and eventually associates with the pain: It reminds him of the pain his mother had always spoken about "*the pain,*" as if a generic term of its own. He then concludes that pain is a thoroughly feminine attribute, which he consequently attributes to the femininity within himself. Here is the dream:

He is in a hospital ward run by a doctor who is none other than Madeleine (his wife). She shows him how to examine a sick person's body. Then he is faced with performing a proctological examination on a man. The man squats in a position as if in Mohammedan prayer (leaning over to the front). His anus is spread wide open by a metal tube that looks to be "at least five times larger in diameter than an anoscope." To examine the anus, Mr. Garance must move in closer, but his vision becomes blurred, he feels dizzy, he cannot see anything in the tube. He has to insert a thin glass pipette into the tube, like those used to draw wine samples from the barrel. The pipette must not break! His hands begin to tremble.

Then he has to remove the metal tube that is dilating the anus. But the sphincter is so tense that this becomes difficult and dangerous because one must not cause a muscle tear when pulling it out. It's similar to pulling a tire off the rim, in small increments. He works his way forward, letting the sphincter rim roll gradually. This resembles the difficulties an obstetrician encounters when pulling the newborn's head out of the vulva without tearing it (note the concept of rebirth that accompanied his hospital stay).

He first associates the color of wine in the pipette with the color of blood. It's difficult to know in this whole scene what is feminine and what is masculine, he says; the pipette, of course, infiltrates and penetrates, but also has the function of pumping – of "blowing," or "pipetting" (in French, these terms are similar: *piper* and *pipeter*).

The image of giving birth through the anus also comes to mind, perhaps like a difficult birth where metal instruments (forceps) must be employed.

His associations then go to from the dream to something he had read previously on the subject of femininity. He is reminded of a film about Françoise Dolto he saw on television. And, finally, he references a text he read in my volume *L'indifférence des sexes,* containing a chapter in which I talk about the smallest muscle that can be stretched. The image of fisting comes to mind. He has, he believes, heard of sexual practices of this nature that lead to the de-differentiation of the sexes.

What we are witnessing here is the remaking of involvement in anal manipulation in the form of expressive acting (*agir expressif*), which is essentially designed to mix the elements of anus, blood, the risks of anal muscle tears, manual manipulation, and finally gazing through a kind of speculum to evoke the blood. This occurs in the wake of the dizziness spell he had experienced just a few weeks earlier, now completely reabsorbed. The "seeing," the blood, the eyes of the red-headed, red-pupiled woman, the other red-headed woman who can be looked at but not touched …

From the vantage point of psychoanalytic working through, the *body's participation* in dreams is essential. In gestures that express voyeurism and sadism, these body games – which in the past had been enough to trigger a somatic crisis when approached purely phantasmatically – are reintegrated or reappropriated thanks to "working through the dream." This working through metabolizes the somatic and delirious decompensation by expanding the expressive registers of the body. Thus, it seems to me, part of what was proscribed in the state of the amential unconscious can be repatriated into the repressed sexual unconscious. This hypothesis admittedly ascribes to the dream a truly transformative capacity that goes beyond what Freud said about dreamwork. The gist lies in the translational function of the dream. According to Laplanche (2017b), Freud rejects the very existence of such a function. For him, dreamwork is the effort expended to produce the dream – and only for this production. In what I present here, however, dreamwork has another function: Thanks to formal regression, dreamwork can provide psychic content with a visual form – content that was previously unrepresented and unsymbolized – by mobilizing the body as represented in the dream by specific actions. These actions take place in the realm for which I have proposed the term "expressive acting out" (*agir expressif*). The latter describes how the body participates in expressing an affect when it is addressed to the other (namely, to the other who, in the basic anthropological situation, is the adult); that is, in the child's attempt, through bodily movements (facial expressions, gestures, psychomotor activity), to signal an impulse they wish to share with the adult. The erotic dimension of this expressive action may trigger in the adult, as if out of compulsion, a reaction to the child's body: "accident of seduction." In this case, the body-play the child tries to establish with the adult is excluded ("proscribed") from the child's communication with the adult – the expressive acting. The latter, however, cannot bear to participate in this game – for reasons stemming from their own unconscious. The game of libidinous subversion – which organizes the emergence of the second, the erogenous body, and whose proscription consequently severely curtails the emergence of the second body in the child – would emerge for the first time in the expressive acting produced qua dreamwork. In the case of Mr. Garance, this play concerns the desire to observe – the voyeuristic play with the adult's body. The dream enables this body-play to take place for the first time.

So, what mobilizes this function of working through expressive acting via the dream? In my opinion, the same thing that sets in motion the transference of sexual drive repertoire in the patient: The latent contents mobilized during the analytic session, in this case, his voyeuristic sexual curiosity for body-play around the anus (of the adult other = the analyst), which arguably come to the surface via his dreamwork in the night following the session. Thus, the "working through" of the experience of sexual arousal in the body was experienced and put into latency during the session.

Such working through, if it occurs, leaves very strong, very vivid impressions upon awakening; the patient remembers such dreams with extreme precision, traces of which remain very sharply etched in pleasant colors in memory. The latter is related to what the dream event induces in the patient: heightened sensations, a surge of expressive bodily registers. Such an expansion of the body's capabilities, experienced like a burst of new pleasure, marks a burgeoning of subjectivity.

The analyst, in turn, should be content to confirm the emergence of a new means of expression. "Yes, it is not uninteresting to look into an asshole."

The neurological disorder abated completely within a few weeks. Analysis continued for another 5 years. Relapse never occurred (to my knowledge).

Conclusion

I based this article on a clinical history of decompensation in a patient who had been in psychoanalysis for several years. The decompensation was accompanied by a somatic crisis (labyrinth neuritis) and a psychotic crisis (delusions). The metapsychological analysis of this decompensation implies a deviation from the psychosomatic theory advocated by the Paris psychosomatic school (Marty & de M'Uzan, 1963).

The main deviation concerns the need to consider not only what happens at the level of psychosomatic economy, not only what is at play at the level of psychological conflict, but also what happens at the level of bodily experience. Locating what happens in the body implies introducing a theory of the body. And just such a metapsychology of the body is the focus of this article. The processes in question concern not only the biological body, but also the experienced body, the latter also referred to by the terms "subjective body" or "erotic body." And then, it is useful to specify how the erotic body functions within the relationship between the child and the (adult) other based on the biological body. To explain this construction, I suggest the concept of a *"libidinous subversion"* of the physiological order in favor of the erotic order, which enables the formation of a second body, the erotic body – the inhabited body – which is the *conditio sine qua non* for being able to experience affects. The second body does not exist from birth; rather, it emerges from the relationship between the child and the (adult) other through the games that occur between the two concerning personal hygiene. I have analyzed these games between the child's body and the adult's body using the general theory of seduction proposed by Jean Laplanche, which insists in particular on the inevitable participation of the adult's sexual unconscious in such interactions with the child. Normally, during body care, the adult's drives remain at a level tolerable to the child ("well-tempered seduction"), allowing libidinous subversion to play its role in the formation of the erotic body and infantile sexuality on the part of the child. In some cases, however, the adult fails to control their arousal (resulting in sexual abuse or violence against the child's body), which ruptures the aura of "well-tempered seduction" and generates an "accident of seduction." The latter, in turn, leads to "fractures" in the development of the child's erotic body, creating zones of fragility in the child's sexual economy.

These "fractures" lie behind the body's "uninhabitable zones" – in other words, the proscribed registers of erotic life that inscribe their harmful traces in the formation of an unconscious sector separate from the repressed sexual unconscious: A split between the two unconscious realms. Can these uninhabitable zones of the body, which have escaped libidinous subversion and deprived the patient of a psychoaffective life, be reclaimed through analytic treatment? Yes, but this would, first of all, require changes in how the psychoanalyst listens and intervenes. It would mean focusing on a particular technique of analyzing "dreamwork," something we call "working through (the scission) by working through the dream."

Notes

1 "Body Worlds" by Von Hagens, see Francis Martens, 2008: La Libre Belgique, 18 September 2008: "Barnum de cadavres." This exhibition links inspection, death, blood, and "no touching."
2 I use the term "translational" for the French neologism "traductif" created by Laplanche.
3 I should point out this does not mean that I subscribe to Freud's phase-oriented conception. I do not adhere to piling up the phases like some evolutionary stratification leading toward a sort of genital and heterosexual maturity. Rather, we are witness to an increase in space, leading to the formation of a "geography," namely, that of the erogenous body.

References

Anzieu, D. (1985): *Das Haut-Ich*. Trans. by M. Korte u. M.-H. Lebourdais-Weiss. Frankfurt a.M.: Suhrkamp.
de Biran, M. (1995 [1807]): "De l'aperception immédiate." In: *Œuvres, Tome IV*. Paris: Editions Vrin.
Dejours, C. (2004): Les meurtrissures du corps. Vortrag im Rahmen der *Entretiens de l'APF* am 5. Juni. *Documents et Débats*, 64, 26–39.
Ferenczi S. (2004 [1932]): Sprachverwirrung zwischen den Erwachsenen und dem Kind. Die Sprache der Zärtlichkeit und der Leidenschaft. In: *Schriften zur Psychoanalyse II*. Gießen: Psychosozial, 303–313.
Freud, S. (1905d): Three Essays on the Theory of Sexuality SE VII, 123–246.
Freud, S. (1915c): Instincts and their Vicissitudes. SE XIV, 109–140.
Freud, S. (1923b): The Ego and the Id. SE XIX, 1–66
Laplanche, J. (1997): The Theory of Seduction and the Problem of the Other. *Int J Psychoanal*, 78, 653–666.
Laplanche, J. (2011 [1987]): *Neue Grundlagen für die Psychoanalyse*. Gießen: Psychosozial.
Laplanche, J. (2017a [1992]): Implantation, Intromission. In: Laplanche, J.: *Die unvollendete kopernikanische Revolution in der Psychoanalyse*. Frankfurt a. M.: Fischer, 109–114.
Laplanche, J. (2017b [2003]): Traum und Mitteilung: Muss man das siebte Kapitel neu schreiben? In: Laplanche, J.: *Sexual. Eine im Freud'schen Sinne erweiterte Sexualtheorie*. Gießen: Psychosozial, 53–75.
Laplanche, J. (2017d [2007]): Inzest und infantile Sexualität. In: Laplanche, J.: *Sexual. Eine im Freud'schen Sinne erweiterte Sexualtheorie*. Gießen: Psychosozial, 245–259.
Marty, P. (1968): La dépression essentielle. *Revue Française de Psychanalyse*, 32, 594–599.
Marty, P., Fain, M. & de M'Uzan, M. (1963): La pensée opératoire. *Revue Française de Psychanalyse*, 27, 345–356.
Marty, P., Fain, M., de M'Uzan, M. & David, C. (1968): Le cas Dora et le point de vue psychosomatique. *Revue Française de Psychanalyse*, 32, 679–685.
Torok, M. (1978): Maladie du deuil et fantasme du cadavre exquis. In: Abraham, N. (Ed.): *L'écorce et le noyau*. Paris: Aubier-Flammarion, 229–251.

Chapter 6

Affect Dialog, Affect Debris, and Encapsulated Body Engrams

Some Reflections on Psychoanalytic Technique with the Bodily Encoded Unconscious

Sebastian Leikert

Introduction

Psychoanalysis has traditionally conceptualized the body as an enigmatic place where vitality and intentionality arise, while at the same time preferring to skip its existence in its modeling and treatment techniques. Currently, perhaps because of the increase of somatic pathologies in our treatment rooms, psychoanalysis has begun to fill this gap (Knoblauch, 2019; Lombardi, 2017; Plassmann, 2019; Tsolas & Anzieu-Premmereur, 2018). I myself proposed models of the *sensual self* and the *encapsulated body engram* (Leikert, 2019) in an effort to move both theory and treatment more toward the level of corporeality. In this chapter, I would like to develop these thoughts from the perspective of affect dialog and its possible failure. Affect dialog denotes the exchange of emotions and affect signals beginning as early as birth and leading to the development of a core psychic structure. It thus describes the sensual self in interaction.

Affect is described here as a performance comprising two components: An affect (such as the joy of being reunited with someone) is composed of an *affect signal*, which communicates the subject's momentary intention and state (such as a welcoming smile and opened arms), and the *activation pattern*, the physical side of the affect (preparing the organism for the affective action). In the case of reunion joy, it is a relaxed and vitalizing activation.

However, a failure of the affect dialog inhibits the expression of the affect and dissociates it from the corresponding activation pattern: The affect signal can no longer be transmitted from the failed affect dialog. Using the above-mentioned example of the joy of reunion, let us imagine what might occur if, contrary to expectation, the joy of being reunited with someone meets with cold rejection on the other person's part, the welcoming smile freezes, the arms sink, and maybe even a feeling of shame ensues. This triggers a completely different activation pattern: Blood flows to the face, creating a blush of shame, an involuntary sign of an affect. Most importantly, affect expression tends to be inhibited because the emotional interaction occurs so

DOI: 10.4324/9781003370130-6

unexpectedly and is, at least momentarily, incomprehensible. Even if the unpleasant feeling is not immediately exhibited, especially in the case of shame – where after all, the affect dialog should be interrupted – it remains in the body-self and partially disorganizes it.

A single interaction like the one described does not lead to pathological structures and a gap in self-organization. Initially, all elements are still accessible to consciousness and self-awareness. However, should such ruptures in affect dialog occur persistently and particularly at a stage of life when self-organization is still immature and fragile, then cumulative traumatization occurs (Masud Khan, 1977 [1963]): The inhibitory processes involved become anchored before the threshold of consciousness and become chronic. The bodily affect impulse is no longer processed, either scenically, in dream sequences, or verbally. Rather, the debris of the failed affect dialog remains in the body-self in the form of disorganized activation patterns. That is what I have come to call *encapsulated body engrams:* the emergence of a physically encoded unconscious.

From the perspective of this conception, a breach occurs between the symbolized unconscious and the encapsulated, bodily encoded unconscious. This breach explains why conventional treatment techniques fail to adequately address the bodily encoded unconscious, which relies on dream imagery, fantasies, and verbalization (Bucci, 1997; Dejours, 2001). But how should we best recalibrate the elements of a psychoanalytic treatment technique (free association, evenly suspended attention, interpretation) to include the bodily encoded unconscious?

This contribution presents a treatment technique that includes just that – the bodily encoded unconscious. It addresses and transforms the body level by implementing a perceptual rather than an interpretive process. In this context, perception is presented as an inherently analytic activity: Perception perceives differences, unraveling through visualization what was previously welded together, conflated, and enmeshed. Body-centered psychoanalytic perceptual work dissolves the repetition compulsions imposed by deeply ingrained habits and allows new connections to arise, both within the body-self and between the body-self and imaginative representations (Leikert, 2023).

I illustrate this treatment technique using a clinical vignette, beginning with a dream in which the failure to symbolize affect emerges. Then, I describe a therapeutic collaboration that aims not at interpreting dream elements but at perceptually exploring and restructuring the body-self, where the debris of primary affect dialog has been stored.

Affect Dialog and Its Breakdown

In this contribution, affect dialog denotes the primary language of communication and relatedness. It comprises the exchange of phonetic and gesticulatory signals, their imitative appropriation, and their development into a primary structure, enabling patterns of emotional signaling and patterns of bodily activation to be grounded and rehearsed. This system of communication, identity, and relatedness is fully functional even before language acquisition. It continues to become ever more differentiated throughout life, parallel to the verbal communication system. At the same time, the affect dialog provides the basic material sublimated in the arts. For example, the emotional valence of prosody – its rhythm and its repetitive patterns – forms the basic material from which music emerges. Regularization of its rhythms gives rise to the meter of music; pitch differences become defined musical intervals and form the basis for both melody and harmony (Leikert, 2017).

Affects are entities consisting of an affect signal and an activation pattern. They communicate states of the organism, such as hunger, readiness to play, anger, or desire for attachment. It is important to understand the diversity of the two parts of the affective whole: The affect signal and the parallel bodily activation pattern represent not only external and internal aspects of the affective event, but they also function according to different laws.

Affects describe the existential relationships the subject maintains with their environment: Joy reflects the desire to take up or deepen a bond; the desire to play characterizes the interest one has in the Other, in the world, and in one's own psychic growth; anger describes the state of self-assertion in a real or psychically dangerous situation. Let us now look at the two sides of the affective event and the different rules they are subject to.

The affective signal of joy is the smile, accompanied by a characteristic facial expression and a soft melodious timbre, tending toward a higher voice register. The corresponding physical activation is a relaxed but involved body. Curiosity lacks a characteristic gesticulatory pattern: It directs all psychic attention toward the object and readies itself to receive and engage with the incoming elements. Once again, an activated but relaxed openness is the reigning bodily pattern. Anger, in contrast, with its increased release of adrenaline and activation of skeletal muscles, projects a very different pattern of bodily activation from the outset. The voice tends to be deeper, complemented by the characteristically different pattern of facial expressions (Krause, 2012).

So, why is it so important to keep the two sides of this whole separate when they would seem to occur in such intimately intertwined ways? First, we are dealing here with the interweaving of different orders and directions of perception: *external* perception and *internal* perception function according to different rules. Second, and even more important, the functional unit of affect breaks down when the dialog of affect fails; the dissociation of these two aspects has yet to be fully grasped by psychoanalytic theory in its systematic weighting of theory and treatment technique.

The Affect Signal and the Gestalt Laws

The affect signal is understood only when it presents itself to the other as a clearly readable gesture or phonetic gestalt. By recognizing the affect, the subject reveals their competence in decoding the meaning of a gestalt. Gestalt laws are the laws of perception. Gestalt imprints itself on the memory and forms the basis for a figurative-scenic memory.

Gestalt psychology explored this level of psychic functioning, originally by von Ehrenfels (1890). Psychoanalysis summarizes these regularities in formulations such as "thinking in pictures" (Freud, 1923b, p. 248), "scenic understanding" (Lorenzer, 1973), or the "imaginary" (Lacan, 1975). It accurately delineates an understanding of image and scene from the function of language, though it does not systematically examine the structural laws of sensory discourse in great detail.

My investigations of esthetics (Leikert, 2017) have examined these structural laws extensively. Here, it suffices to refer, on the one hand, to the gestalt organization of the perceptual and pictorial levels and, on the other hand, to emphasize that repetition and ritualization play major roles. The affect signal is received via the external senses and functions according to gestalt laws.

A vocal statement conveys the emotional message through volume, a hardness or softness of the voice, and a melodic or abrasive tone. The laws of gestalt in music, perceived through clear rules of repetition, also regulate the expression of the vocal timbre. Likewise, the visual expression is most clearly addressed by gestalt-like clear expression patterns. The latter in turn develops further into a pictorial language, the basis of dream life, and finally gives rise to a system of expressing affect and understanding sensory signals. In other words, this process makes a mental apparatus available for mentalizing affect (Schulz-Venrath, 2013, 2021; Stern, 2003 [1985]).

Activation Pattern and the Body-Self – The Dark Side of the Moon

Activation patterns, i.e., the bodily activation that matches the affect, take place in the incomprehensibly complex interplay of cerebral, hormonal, and muscular innervation and inhibition processes. They interconnect to form a whole that shapes our visible physicality and attractiveness. Most importantly, this is where the subject's sense of life emerges. It shapes how someone inhabits their body, whether they experience it as a good place, one of vitality and enjoyment, or, at the other extreme, as a place of catastrophic pain, something to be escaped. The body-self system emerges, which contains the various activation patterns and coordinates (or discoordinates) its actions. The body-self, its motor patterns, and its specific activation profiles that reflect experiences usually remain hidden in the depths of consciousness, standing in the shadow of the clearly visible figures of imaginative (gestalt) or verbal consciousness. The body-self, as a formative world of experience, is simultaneously always present and always concealed: *The dark side of the moon.*

Nevertheless, bodily states and sensations can also become the object of perception at any time. Freud (1923b, p. 21) concedes: "Inner perception yields sensations of processes from the most diverse, certainly also the deepest, layers of the psychic apparatus. They are poorly known; their best pattern can still be considered those of the pleasure-unpleasure array." Psychoanalysis is not in the habit of bringing proprioceptive perceptions to the forefront of attention, and indeed, this is not necessary as long as the integrity of the sensory self is not destroyed by traumatization. But if this should be the case, then we need to find a technique that actively involves this area. Of course, working with the body-self and listening to one's own body resonance are also possible with less disturbed patients (Gendlin, 2014; Ruettner et al., 2015). However, this method is crucial to successful treatment, especially where discoherences and encapsulated engrams have massively damaged the self.

It is essential to realize that the body is part of the psychic landscape, not only in the case of a serious pathology, such as we are examining here, but in every situation that occurs in its activation patterns and psychic activities. Not just the petrified, dulled body of the traumatized individual but also the living, erotic body of the healthy person reflect elements of the psychic structure and form the setting for how they view life (Dejours, 2001, and in this book).

Affects and Their Intersubjective Mediation

We should not approach affects from an individual perspective; they develop in intersubjective space. The development of the sensory self, with a functioning coordination of the affect system and the body-self, depends on good communication in the primary relationship. The mirroring of emotions and the sensitive response to infant needs differentiate the newborn's genetically inherent ability to recognize affects and signal own states. The primary affect dialog lays the foundation for an integrated sensory self-system in which internal and external perception, affect expression, and activation patterns can coordinate. This context requires intersubjective repetition processes and ritualizations. Stern's concept of generalized interactional representations sums this up quite well (Stern, 2003 [1985], p. 143).

The core body-self can only stabilize and communicate within its patterns if it finds sufficient consistency in repetition. Such consistency comes about through rhythm and repetition and strives not only to establish a good connection to the object but also to establish a good coherence within the sensory self, i.e., to coordinate activation patterns and affect signals with each other. Malloch and Trevarthen (2009) use music analogies to show how such repetitive constellations are created and rehearsed in spontaneous rituals between mother and child.

A nursery rhyme such as the *Itsy Bitsy Spider* or lullabies are examples of such microrituals in the mother-child dyad. They strengthen the bond with the mother, while at the same time consolidating the inner coherence of the self; the connection between the body-self and symbolic form is deepened through such little rituals. The affect theme in question here is one of falling and being held in the relationship at the same time (Leikert, 2016). We return to this theme in the context of the clinical vignette.

Affect Debris

Even in a successful coordination process between mother and child, we can always observe some instances when the coordination fails, leading to disruptions and the need for re-regulation (Knoblauch, 2019). But what results when such dysregulations become chronic or remain unresolved? Since the 1970s, researchers have studied such questions using Edward Tronick's so-called "still-face experiment." This method reveals that the baby not only stops all gestural and mimic activity in response to the mother's lack of affect response, but also that all physiological parameters become dysregulated (Weinberg & Tronick, 1996). For ethical reasons, such minitraumatizations by resonance denial are terminated before they can cause permanent damage. However, since Masud Khan's (1963) concept of "cumulative trauma," psychoanalysis has assumed that repeated traumatizations of affect dialog accumulate and leave their mark on a dysregulated body-self (Bucci, 2002; van der Kolk, 2015). Let us consider the situation regarding the subsystems of affect signaling and the body-self.

The above-mentioned still-face experiment is a good way to illustrate these connections. There, the mother of an approximately 1-year-old child is asked to engage first in normal affect dialog with the child, greeting and joking with them, etc. Once the affect dialog has been established, the mother turns away from the child for a moment, then back to the child, but now no longer showing any mimicry or vocal reaction: A still face. The child reacts with multiple attempts to regain the mother's attention and resonance, but then shows increasing desperation upon failing in these attempts, and after a short time loses composure. Before the situation reaches damaging proportions, the mother turns back to the child (Tronick & Cohn, 1989; Tronick, 2007).

This experiment clearly demonstrates how quickly affective signaling stops when the dialog breaks down and the subject is deprived of sensitive resonance by the other. At the same time, the body-self enters a dysregulated state in its activation patterns, which does not just stop but seeks a new balance. Yet that balance may be dysfunctional, and the antagonistic parties may end up reaching a stable compromise in the body-self that no longer serves emotion processing. The two halves of the sensory self – the activation pattern and the affect sign – now proceed to disintegrate, a state I call "affect debris": The integrity of the child's directed somatopsychic intentionality, which addresses the other using gestures and mimicry, falls apart. This means, first of all, that affect signaling comes to a disorganized standstill. This not only destroys any direct affective expressivity, but it also causes the mentalizing ability to translate psychic content into images and scenes to cease – or become ineffective. In this fragile state of self-development, the subject still needs a resonant caregiver to help mentalize their inner states. I refer to this as the "inhibition barrier," following Freud's defense mechanism of inhibition (Freud, 1926d). This defense process causes the traumatic zones of the body-self to be excluded from further processing and psychic growth. The body-self system now becomes the sole carrier of information concerning the traumatic interaction. "Dead zones" form within the body-self (Dejours, 2001), and disorganized configurations within the body-self congeal to create dysfunctional forms of equilibrium.

The image of debris contains the idea of falling: The edifice of the sensual self "falls" to rubble. And indeed, clinically, the experience of falling into the infinite seems to be a specific symptom in the context of early traumatic interruptions of experience (Tustin, 2005, p. 40). Ogden describes the collapse of the sense of self within the earliest psychic organization, the autistic-touching position, as "the skin becoming a sieve through which the interior oozes out and falls into an endless and formless space" (Ogden, 1995 [1989], p. 40). Elsewhere (Leikert, 2021b), I have described working with analysands in whom this experience of falling into nonexistence or vertigo lay at the core of their physical symptomatology. The vignette described below also concerns this process.

Two Steps – From Passivity to Active Processing

Affects are entities consisting of activation patterns and affect signals. A closer look at this duality, however, reveals a significant difference between the two halves in terms of the processing subject: The subject is passive regarding the activation pattern, whereas regarding the affect signal, the subject actively seeks to appropriate this original passivity, shape it, and introduce it into an intersubjective processing process. Modern infant research rightly emphasizes the "competent infant," though this competence concerns the processing of an original passivity, i.e., a state the child did not actively select or generate. Infants do not choose their hunger; hunger arises in them without their input. Infants do not choose their parents or their parents' (un)predictability. Once again, we clearly see this in the still-face experiment: The infant does not create the constellation but is passively subjected to it. The infant's affect signals demonstrate the attempt to competently shape the situation. Yet, the infant's competence quickly reaches its limits, and the responsible adult recognizes the traumatic gravity of this process and aborts it. In our therapy, we deal with inner worlds in which *exactly* this failed to happen, leading to the subsequent accumulation of traces of traumatic events.

The Encapsulated Body Engram, the Disorganized Body-Self

States of traumatic dysregulation in the body-self do not simply disappear when the external situation changes. Because of the inhibition barrier, traces and engrams of these traumatic events remain encapsulated, become isolated in the body-self, and persist dissociated from the fabric of linguistic and pictorial representations. I proposed the term "encapsulated body engrams" for such formations" (Leikert, 2019, 2021a, 2021b, 2023). The term "body engram" emphasizes the passive nature of bodily inscription; Laplanche (1996, p. 109) speaks of "intromission" in this regard. First and foremost, this describes the fact of the child's original passivity in the human encounter. The process becomes problematic through the collapse, the "falling to rubble," of the communicative process, which inhibits the expression of affect and prevents the inscription of experiences in representational systems. Instead, affect is encapsulated in a bodily activation pattern. Laplanche (2017 [2003], p. 178) speaks here of the "complete failure" of translation, i.e., of the impossibility of translating the "enclosed unconscious" (p. 179).

There are two ways to look at this moment of encapsulation: One occurs within the body-self and the other in the representational system that dominates our sense of self. Within the body-self, conspicuous misperceptions indicate dysfunctional patterns of activation. In the clinical example described below, we can identify three types of misperceptions:

- falling as the sensation of no longer being able to reside in one's own body;
- devitalization, paresthesias, and numbness; and
- changes in normal rhythmic regulatory processes, suggesting the experience of stress and threat (rapid breathing, palpitations).

Here, we cannot provide a comprehensive phenomenological review of encapsulated body engrams, but I have described further variants elsewhere (Leikert, 2019).

Because the perception of body-self states does not possess the gestalt clarity of a dream image or verbalization, they are all too easy to overlook. When the analysand describes them, i.e., introduces them into the associative chain, therapists often overlook them because they are recounted using language that psychoanalysis has not yet become accustomed to speaking. Or they are immediately interpreted. Lombardi's (2017) treatment technique of focusing on the dissociation of body and psyche is an example of how to proceed by attempting to include the body's unmentalized signals.

My suggestion, however, goes in a different direction: I encourage my analysands to pay full attention to internal perception over longer periods of time. This enables them, first and foremost, to perceive what is going on in the body-self and what dramas are permanently playing out in the shadow areas of the psyche besides those that emerge in the foreground drama of verbal dialog. We can describe the processes of inhibition and segmentation, dysregulation, and the attempt to return to a constructive state of self-regulation. We are not dealing here with activation patterns of distinctly primary effects but with their fragments – their debris and buried resonances.

If one succeeds in directing perception to the level of proprioception for longer periods of time, one recognizes how the analysand begins to reorganize their body-self within the resonant psychoanalytic dyad. My approach is to enable the long-term anchoring of the analytic process in the dialog from one body-self to the other. The prerequisite for this to succeed is the willingness of the analysand to devote themselves to describing their body perceptions over longer periods of time, as well as the willingness of the analyst to accompany this process with resonant listening, i.e., paying special attention to their body resonances.

Encapsulated body engrams are dissociated from all other psychic life; experiences are not mentalized and fail to be represented by language and images. The affective catastrophes deposited in encapsulated body engrams are missing an adequate connection to symbolic networks (Laplanche, 2017, p. 179) and are, thus, not inscribed in the symbolic coordinates of time. Rather, they remain outside of psychic time and are experienced as a permanent threat. This, in turn, unsettles and undermines the sense of life in the form of an urgent sense of namelessness. To be sure, the fragments of emotional integrity remain effective in their affective valence; at the same time, they are no longer perceptible because affect signaling and scenic memory are missing. Clear and directed emotions such as anger or joy linked to comprehensible memories of the causative event are absent. Instead, unclear misperceptions dominate, which are usually not well differentiated and thus also at risk of slipping under the radar of the standard psychoanalytic technique.

Reaccentuating the Psychoanalytic Treatment Technique

If one approaches the psychoanalytic setting and the elements of the treatment technique with the thoughts developed so far, new aspects ensue. Diagnostically, the question is whether an inhibition barrier and bodily disorganization are at hand or whether a coherent psychic structure is present. Once work has commenced with patients with structural distur-bances and ruptures between their body-self and their representational systems, the previous central treatment technique focused on interpretation should not be chosen, since interpretation inherently links linguistic elements and is based on the assumption that all relevant parts of the psychic organization are – and remain – linked to the linguistic network. That is how one accesses the symbolic unconscious, which is structured in dreams, failures, etc. However, this fails to include dissociated formations and those separated by inhibition processes. Increasingly, therapists are searching for more noninterpretive effective factors of analytic therapy (Stern et al., 2002). Schulz-Venrath, for example, speaks of a "turning away from all forms of interpretive technique that do not enable mentalizing" (Lohmer & Schulz-Venrath, 2020, p. 145). The interpretive technique can be extended to include a technique that trusts the psychoanalytic process to proceed even beyond linguistic networks – oriented solely toward bodily perception.

Psychoanalytic Perception Work as a Supplement to the Technique of Interpretation

But how to anchor the perceptual treatment technique in psychoanalytic theory? How does it relate to the interpretive technique? Must it be imported from other therapeutic directions, or is it grounded in the foundation of the psychoanalytic treatment technique itself?

The psychoanalytic process is set in motion by a basic rule formulated specifically for each of the two partners in the analytic dyad. The analysand employs free association to express everything that presents itself to the inner perception. But the analyst equally follows this principle: Nothing is to be privileged – everything, even apparent trivialities, is given equal attention. Freud repeatedly emphasized that the analyst has to put aside any acquired abilities, any desire to obtain an overview, to prevent disturbing the receptive unconscious in its function by applying preconceived wishes and convictions. In his three concise rules for dealing with dreams, Freud twice warns the analyst not to interrupt the receptive process by forwarding a hasty understanding:

> (1) We must not concern ourselves with what the dream *appears* to tell us [...] (2) We must restrict our work to calling up the substitutive ideas for each element, we must not reflect about them [...] (3) We must wait till the concealed unconscious material we are in search of emerges of its own accord. (Freud, 1916–1917, p. 114)

The central axis of psychoanalytic methodology is based on the function of perception. Psychoanalytic work is first and foremost perceptual work, and pure perception forms the core of the procedure. Perception is the eye in the storm of the analytic process.

Yet, there are many different objects of perception. Freud lists words and images (dream images) as well as feelings, sensations, and bodily perceptions as objects of perception. Although in 1923, he conceded that "little is known" (Freud, 1923b, p. 21) concerning these bodily sensations, he sees no reason to exclude them from the chain of association or psychoanalytic attention. On the contrary, "internal perceptions yield sensations of processes arising in the most diverse and certainly also in the deepest strata of the mental apparatus" (1923b, p. 21).

Thus, the principle of pure, nonprivileged perception generates the principle of equal treatment of the elements of all three levels – bodily sensations (as derivatives of activation patterns), images, and words. If all three systems constitute the subject structure, the treatment technique should ensure that all three areas are included in the analytic process (Plassmann, 2011). In practice, however, word associations clearly lie in the foreground. For this very reason, Freud also privileges the treatment of dream images, which to him represent the royal road to the unconscious in a characteristically different way than the rule of free association would dictate. Here, Freud intervenes in the inter-connections and actively prefers the individually manifested dream elements. In the second of his three rules for dealing with dreams, Freud recommends focusing on dream images: "We must restrict our work to calling up the substitutive ideas for each element" (Freud, 1916–1917, p. 114). Thus, the therapist should not wait to see which associations arise on their own, but rather – according to Freud – focus on the individual elements to make the dream's message – with its fluctuating and fleeting images – accessible to the analytic process.

This focusing principle is also appropriate for dealing with encapsulated body engrams. Both Bucci (1997) and Lombardi (2017) repeatedly emphasize the need to focus on bodily perceptions to process primary defenses and dissociations. Let's take a look at perceptual work with bodily sensations.

The Somatic Narration

We cannot understand the message of a dream by interpreting an isolated, manifest dream element, nor can we understand the message of an encapsulated engram by taking only a brief look at a single bodily sensation. My suggestion is, especially at the beginning of an analytic collaboration, to focus on bodily sensations for a long time and to anchor the analytic process solely in the intercorporeity of the analytic dyad. This is what I call "somatic narration." The analyst supports the analysand in verbalizing their bodily perceptions, thus giving the encapsulated engrams a linguistic representation within the analytic space. Any interspersed interpretations would interrupt the highly precarious process of somatic narration. Bodily sensations link together to form a somatic narrative that we do not, or not yet, understand. Listening to such a somatic narrative with our own thoughts – but especially with our own somatic resonances – has a high curative value (Ruettner et al., 2015; Volz-Boers, 2016).

The structure of human subjectivity consists of three subsystems: The body-self (a system of activation patterns), the level of scene and gestalt (arising from the affect signal), and the verbal-self. Mental health is based on the flexible interconnectedness of these subsystems. However, splitting off (Dejours, 2001) or dissociation (Bucci, 2002; Lombardi, 2017) of central areas of the body-self occurs as part of the defense process. Interpretations during the processing of these formations are not helpful because they remain within the system of the verbal-self. The encapsulated body engram should be worked through at the interbody level of the analytic relationship. The "capsule" can open only from within. Regarding the encapsulated engram, only an analysand's spontaneous contemplations that develop while they work through their bodily sensations are of any value.

The Cartography of the Body Landscape

Yet not only the imaginary elements of contemplation are useful in analytic work: The somatic narrative produces its own outcome. Verbalizing bodily sensations establishes personal and concrete connections between the verbal-self and the body-self. Verbalizing the landscape of bodily sensations creates a map of the body-self with its various craters, chasms, barriers, and incoherences, which now become the property of the verbal memory of the analytic dyad and provide a clear and orienting differentiation of the analysand's relationship to their self. This act of mapping is never forgotten; it accompanies the work of the therapeutic dyad as a means of comparing changes in self-states, and it constitutes a sort of calibration tool. Such verbalization serves the analysand as a new object of self-reference. The map of the body-self created in the psychoanalytic perceptual work is then gradually transferred to the autonomous possession of the analysand, who compares their momentary self-state with previous ones. This enables the analysand to increasingly shift the process of visualizing and working-through states of the body-self into the realm of autonomous ego functions.

Clinical Vignette

In the following clinical vignette, I report on work with an analysand who was already quite advanced. The unconscious theme of falling out of a relationship was no longer represented solely by bodily feelings and encapsulated engrams, but the dream function had already begun to symbolize physically encoded states of suffering through dream imagery. The theme was both bodily and symbolically encoded. Elsewhere, I have described treatments in which the encapsulated engrams first had to be worked through before dreams could be addressed (Leikert, 2021a, 2021b). This vignette describes a later phase in the analytic work, where both forms of representation are mixed.

The session described took place during the third year of analysis with Mr. T., who had originally consulted me during a serious life crisis in which he felt he was losing all orientation. In the past, various severe depressive episodes and depersonalization states had been treated by inpatient psychiatric care, albeit without lasting success. From about the second year of analysis on, we repeatedly worked with bodily sensations, exploring and resolving massive feelings of being a stranger in one's own body.

In the phase in which the described session originated, Mr. T. was experiencing a depressive crisis; he felt powerless, was on sick leave from work, and lacked the energy to care for himself or to communicate with his partner. During this session, he reported these feelings and then described a dream.

Mr. T:	I am on an upper floor of a high-rise building, with stairs and hallways. There is a big hole in the middle of the hallway, and several people are there. I am lying very close to the hole. There is no railing, and I am afraid of falling down the hole. My father is also there, lying close to me. He says I shouldn't be afraid, but I am afraid. Then another scene comes. People are on a bridge. Among them is Anne Frank. Someone bumps into her and she falls off the bridge. But no one takes any notice. Another scene: Mother is making liverwurst sandwiches. But she's so far away, she doesn't notice any of this.
Me:	*The analytic relationship was familiar and supportive. Mr. T. had already gone through several crises, and I was optimistic that, this time, too, there was no threat of a complete crash. The dream captivated and electrified me immediately; I had the feeling that I could interpret it. We had often talked about the fact that he had not felt securely held by his mother. In regular bouts of binge eating, Mr. T. had tried to assuage these feelings of emptiness and inner lack of support. The element of falling was dominant in the dream-like images that developed in me. It was as if I were lying on an inclined plane and sliding toward the hole in the hallway. I also intensely felt the fall of Anne Frank with great vividness. Kinetic associations (experience of movement) arose in me alongside mental ideas. At the same time, I perceived Mr. T.'s fear and tension. I first asked him about his affects, to determine the intensity of his tension.*
Me:	How do you feel right now?
Mr. T:	I feel tense and shaky.
Me:	*I was having my own vivid kinetic body associations. Mr. T. used the word "shaky," which is authentic and not so generic as "anxious." I concluded that his underlying*

	bodily experience might become accessible and directed my attention to the body.
Me:	What other bodily perceptions are you having?
Mr. T:	Everything is still. There's a tightness, like I'm resisting a feeling. It's like there's a hinge between my head and my body. I seem to be pressing my head into the couch to help me hold on. I know I have legs, but I can't feel them. I can feel my chest, yes, but nothing further down.
Me:	Yes …
Mr. T. *(after 3minutes):*	I can barely breathe. My heart is pounding hard from fear. I'm afraid of falling. Everything around me is contracting. I'm becoming small inside, like a pin. Only a kernel or pit remains. It can make itself small enough to avoid falling down. It's as if I'm crawling into myself.
Me:	Yes …
Mr. T. *(after 5 minutes):*	My breathing is getting faster now. I can control it. The pressure is receding. Now, I feel I can fall asleep.
Me:	Aha, the anxiety is less now?
Mr. T:	Yes, the anxiety has lessened. But my body is not there yet. I can feel my chest breathing, moving. My forehead feels heavy; my eyes are pushed inward. It's about to explode. My butt feels ghost-like, like a phantom pain, but in reverse. People with phantom pain have pain where there is no longer a body part, yet they have pain. I know my butt and leg are there, but I can't feel them. I try to extend my nerves there, but no signal comes back.
Me:	Aha … so, it's like you're trying to regain feeling, in the butt and the legs.
Mr. T. *(after 3 minutes):*	Yes. Now my head feels loose, as if it is not connected to the body. The signal is too weak. As if cut off. Just move! But I can't. Like in a magic show: A man lies down in a box, plates are pushed in, and the box is pushed apart, and there is no connection.
Me:	*I continued to silently accompany this self-exploration, to grasp the images. When I thought about the image of the magic show, I recalled how incredulously I myself had watched such performances as a child, fascinated and frightened at the same time, although of course I knew that no one was really being cut in half. I had the impression that Mr. T. needed no help from me and had fully arrived at the point of intense body exploration. I continued to listen.*
Me:	Hmm …

Mr. T. (after 2 minutes):	My neck is now so tense it hurts. (Pause) Now I feel my leg. It's like an electric shock. As if the line is now free, which almost hurts, this electric shock. Now the other leg, as if an anvil on top of it. A heavy weight.
Me:	*I accompanied the report with my own associations of a primarily kinetic nature. Suddenly, the memory of an acupuncture treatment session surfaced in me, where the doctor's needle sent a kind of electric shock from my foot through my leg.*
Mr. T. (after 5 minutes):	Now everything is heavy. I lie flat and heavy on the couch. I say: Why don't you just move? But I can't move.
Me:	Okay, follow this impulse. We're near the end of the hour now, and I think you need a little time to get back to everyday life.
Mr. T:	Yes, but that is easier said than done. The magician hasn't taken the plates out yet. (Mr. T. then moves, stretching his limbs and rubbing his hands). It feels like I've done some heavy muscle training. Is the hour over already? It can't be! The time just flew by! Now I actually feel looser. I want to shake it all out. Everything is lighter now, and I feel relieved. It's funny to say that, but I feel lighter … relieved.
Me:	*I observed that Mr. T. chose his words from bodily feelings: The perception, "everything is lighter now" leads to the word "relieved." The connection between body and verbalization has been restored.*
Me:	Ah, so you feel physically lighter?
Mr. T:	Yes, somehow relieved.
Me:	That's all for today, I'll see you again next week.

Discussion

The affective center of Mr. T.'s dream is the feeling of falling. I interpret the sensation of being dropped, of falling without being caught, as a somatized memory of traumatic ruptures in the primary affective dialog with his mother.

The phenomenology of falling, especially falling without being caught, is familiar from the psychopathology of early disorders and psychoses (Ogden, 1995 [1989]; Schreber, 1973 [1903]). It seems helpful to me that Winnicott's notion that the fear of going crazy, i.e., of falling out of the web of the symbolized, reflects the memory of early catastrophes (Winnicott, 2018) – of falling into disarray ("falls to rubble," see above) during the primary affect dialog. This memory is deposited in encapsulated engrams or, as in this case, in an experience that refers to the body in its entirety, i.e., to the agonizing feeling of being a stranger in one's own body.

But let us consider the treatment decision I made. I decided against the Freudian method of calling for associations, i.e., further ideas and images. My reason lay primarily in the observation that this session had enabled crucial access to the structures of the patient's body-self. This stemmed not only from the symbolic dream material and the specific affectivity of Mr. T., but also from the positive kinetic reactions on my part. This session had permitted communication from body-self to body-self:

> By means of an isomorphic format we can map [...] others' emotions and sensations onto our own viscereomotor and somatosensory representations. (Lemma, 2015, p. 15)

I had followed my conviction that we would have missed an opportunity had we worked with the dream images at that moment. One could also say that I chose to work with the analysand to address the dark sides of the dream images, those structures of the body-self that usually lie in the shadows.

Undoubtedly: Mr. T. was able to symbolize the failure of symbolization. I could have interpreted this, but then I would have missed the rare opportunity to access the body-self's activation patterns. I was convinced that the images would still be remembered in the next session. However, working with bodily sensations and working through encapsulated engrams can succeed only at the very moment of their occurrence; one cannot actively address them any more than one could ask the analysand to dream a dream. The gateway to such work is always a bodily paresthesia, urgently reported in the here and now of the analytic session.

My decision to focus perception on the region of bodily engrams enabled us to examine the disorganized activation patterns and work through them. Such descriptions form the basis for a differentiated phenomenology of typical constellations of physically organized defenses: the segmentation of the body, the interruption of the connection between head and torso, the paresthesias in the legs, the flattening and control of the breath, and the experience of shrinking and virtually disappearing into one's own body. All of these comprise the vocabulary of the disorganized body-self.

Let us consider what happens during the process of working through bodily sensations. The feeling of falling is present in the act of being condensed to a single point in one's own body. The individual elements of the narrative – the numbness in the legs, the electric shock sent through the limbs, and the body's segmentation (image of the magician cutting up the body) – are enigmatic; they do not fit together like a puzzle, as Freud contended for dream interpretation. While the therapist might resort to an interpretive perspective, my experience is that cautious understanding and mere resonant accompaniment better serve the analysand to improve their mentalizing skills.

This form of psychoanalytic collaboration requires a high tolerance for "not knowing." The elements of somatic narration can sometimes be assigned to concrete biographical situations; much more often, however, they are and remain heuristically useless: They remain inscrutable. On the other hand, they clearly represent elements of a process that leads from fragmentation to self-regulation, from dissociation to interconnectedness. The description above of my own stream of images as well as bodily experienced notions makes it clear that the process of working through sensations is realized in both participants of the analytic dyad. The analyst's interior is populated by a mixture of mental deliberations, clinical decisions, graphic ideas, and kinetic impulses.

During the working through of these zones, the analyst's attentive perception of their own corporeality seems to me to fulfill a central role in the containing process. Again, it is important to note that the work takes place outside of familiar heuristic waypoints. What is the hidden meaning behind my bodily associations with the acupuncture treatment? It remains a mystery. It seems reasonable to me to assume that, in such moments of imitative mirror responses, the two bodies in the analytic dyad are engaged in an intense exchange and containment that is elusive to a linguistic reflection of any particulars. A previously shattered intermediate corporeality is established once again. One can also describe the encapsulated engrams as the collapse of intercorporeity.

Even if the processes remain elusive to the analysand as well, the analysand does perceive the willingness of the analyst to share an experience. "The analyst must operate on the same unorganized levels of fluid, untranslatable, and potentially explosive sensations that the analysand is living through" (Lombardi, 2017, p. 35). Working through archaic fears at the original site of disorganized activation patterns and filling in the gap in the symbolization of these fears of annihilation belongs to this process.

Let us now turn to the interconnectedness between the body-self and the heuristically accessible image plane. I decided to postpone the Freudian approach until the next session, which then revolved around classifying and further contextualizing what I had experienced. In this session, Mr. T. reported that, in the car on the way home from the last session, he had envisioned making himself smaller in his own body: It had brought to mind the image of an embryo without an umbilical cord – that was how he had felt. Indeed, this was a poignant image of being essentially at the mercy of others and of experiencing a lack of contact in the maternal relationship. Mr. T.'s second idea referred to the dream material in a narrower sense: He urgently wanted to report an association that had occurred to him regarding the dream content in which Anne Frank was pushed off the bridge. It was quite simple, he said: As a homosexual, he too would have been gassed by the Nazis. Again, the fear of annihilation was a distinct part of the dream.

The sensation of falling embodies an archaic fear (Tustin, 2005; Winnicott, 2018). To overcome trauma from the primary relationship, one must necessarily work through it thoroughly. The locus lies in bodily sensations, the center of focus in the working-through process. The experience of falling results from a failed sensual dialog in which the feeling of being held securely (primordial trust) failed to materialize at the primary bodily level. The bodily unconscious thus becomes fixed to this tormenting relational figure. Since such a relational figure is present only subsymbolically in the body, there is a constant feeling of existential insecurity, even if secondary formations – such as linguistic or mathematical abilities – are impressively well developed as overcompensation. The archaic relational figure involves a malignant fusioning with a primary object that not only fails to provide security but also threatens abandonment. According to Winnicott, such people know very well what it means *not* to be held securely, "They know what it is like to be dropped, to fall forever, or to become split into psychosomatic disunion" (Winnicott, 1989 [1969], p. 259). Such a fall is experienced as a threat of complete annihilation, which corresponds to the fear of being unable to survive separation from the malignant mother introject. However, if one can work through these fears via transference and countertransference, the fall can finally be realized cathartically and experienced as a liberating separation. Several processes now take place in parallel: The body-self gains coherence by working through moments of disorganization; it can detach itself from the malignant fusion; and now, for the first time, it can inaugurate mature contact with later acquired structures. The previous secondary self-structures, established as compensation, become connected with the coherent body-self. New stability of the self is experienced.

The session described above proved to be a turning point in the analysis. While we had previously addressed elements of the analysand's feelings of persecution and annihilation, only at this point did the sensation of falling – the source of his absolute fear of annihilation – become symbolized and dreamed. Before, Mr. T. had always experienced tensions at work as forebodings of annihilation. Even small disagreements culminated in powerlessness, anxiety, and the need for sick leave. Suddenly, however, arguments at work became something Mr. T. could enjoy: "I didn't know arguing could be such fun."

Similarly, Mr. T. could now afford to break certain rules. He reported that, to shorten his way to work, he had come to drive the wrong way through one-way streets, which precipitated astonishment and disbelief in his partner, since he had previously experienced Mr. T. as decidedly timid. Before, absolute obedience to rules had been necessary to keep his intense fears of annihilation in check.

Mr. T. reported all these changes in the session that followed our body-oriented working through of the dream. The basal instability of his self-experience has not since reappeared.

Concluding Remarks

Affects are not simple psychological entities; an affect is a phenomenon that lies at the center of multiple interactions. First, it consists of two heterogeneous entities, the bodily activation pattern and the affect signal, which must properly interact to ensure good affect processing. Affective patterns also emerge in the intersubjective dialog: They develop in an emotionally differentiated, resonant environment and become the central means of processing experience and social communication. In nonresonant or toxic relationships, on the other hand, multiple processes occur that impoverish the interplay of activation patterns and affect signals, causing the body-self to become increasingly disconnected from the process of experience processing. Experience is in danger of flattening or becoming disorganized.

If traumatizing relationship catastrophes do occur, the affect dialog falls into ruins, and the affect signal is completely cut off, while encapsulated engrams are formed in the body-self; the relationship catastrophe is now frozen in time and lacks all means of expression. The catastrophe cannot be experienced and processed but lurks as a silent and nameless threat beyond the reach of more mature representational systems.

During psychoanalytic treatment, the first step is to assess the presence of emotional resonance processes, whether inhibited or split off. In all preoedipal disorders, the analyst can assume that emotion inhibition and dissociation lie at the root of difficulties in processing experiences and psychic integration. In these situations, the analyst should make an effort to establish a perceptive and receptive attitude in the analytic dialog.

If the analyst has the impression that essential parts of the core-self are separated from mental growth by processes of encapsulation, and that the ability to mentalize is severely limited, they must consider this when applying the treatment technique. The analyst should try to focus on the disruptions in the networks of psychic representational formation and body experience. Only when the connection between body-self and symbolic representation has once again become largely functional can productive interpretive work be done.

Research on the notion of purposefully including such ruptures in therapy is still in its early stages. Wherever the opportunity arises to work with body perceptions over longer periods of time – thus enabling the mapping of a fractured or inhibited body-self – a body-emotionally resonant dyad can take up the task of analytically working through these fractures. This demands that the analyst patiently listen to the somatic narrative and be willing to work outside of the usual heuristic practices. However, working through encapsulated bodily engrams usually results in a discernible gain in emotional accessibility and psychic coherence.

References

Bucci, W. (1997): Symptoms and symbols: A multiple code theory of somatization. *Psychoanal Inq*, 17(2), 151–172.

Bucci, W. (2002): The referential process, consciousness, and the sense of self. *Psychoanal Inq*, 22(5), 766–793. DOI:10.1080/07351692209349017

Dejours, C. (2001): *Le corps d'abord – Corps biologique, Corps érotique et sens moral*. Paris: Payot.

v. Ehrenfels, C. (1890): Über Gestaltqualitäten. *Vierteljahrsschrift für wissenschaftliche Philosophie*, 14, 249–292.

Freud, S. (1916–1917): Introductory Lectures on Psycho-Analysis. SE XV 1-240

Freud, S. (1923b): The Ego and the Id. SE XIX, 1–66

Freud, S. (1926d): Inhibitions, Symptoms and Anxiety. SE XX, 75–176

Gendlin, E. T. (2014): *Focusing – Selbsthilfe bei der Lösung persönlicher Probleme*. Reinbek: Rowohlt.

Knoblauch, S. H. (2019): Fluidität der Emotionen und Verletzlichkeit in der therapeutischen Situation. *Psyche – Z Psychoanal*, 73, 235–263.

Krause, R. (2012): *Allgemeine psychodynamische Behandlung- und Krankheitslehre*. Stuttgart: Kohlhammer.

Lacan, J. (1975): *Schriften*. Olten: Walter.

Laplanche, J. (1996): *Die unvollendete kopernikanische Revolution in der Psychoanalyse*. Frankfurt a. M.: Fischer.

Laplanche, J. (2017 [2003]): *Sexual – Eine im Freud'schen Sinne erweiterte Sexualtheorie*. Gießen: Psychosozial.

Leikert, S. (2017): "For beauty is nothing but the beginning of terror ..." – the outlining of a general psychoanalytic aesthetic. *IJP*, 98, 3, 657–681.

Leikert, S. (2016): Musik, Affektregulation und die Fähigkeit, für sich zu sein – Überlegungen zur Bedeutung der Musik in biographischen Schwellensituationen. *KJP*, 170, 185–203.

Leikert, S. (2019): *Das sinnliche Selbst. Das Körpergedächtnis in der psychoanalytischen Behandlungstechnik*. Frankfurt a. M.: Brandes & Apsel.

Leikert, S. (2021a): Verkapselte Körperengramme und die Traumfunktion – Zur Bearbeitung primärer Abwehrprozesse im Körperselbst. *Forum Psychoanal*. 10.1007/s00451-021-00425-w

Leikert, S. (2021b): Encapsulated body engrams and somatic narration – Integrating body memory into psychoanalytic technique. *Int J Psychoanal*, 102(4), 671–688. 10.1080/00207578.2021.1927044

Leikert, S. (2023) Unrepresented states and the bodily unconscious. *Psychoanalytic Quarterly*, 92(1), 59–81, https://doi.org/10.1080/00332828.2023.2178167

Lemma, A. (2015): *Minding the body. The body in psychoanalysis and beyond*. London: Routledge. Dtsch.

Lohmer, M. & Schulz-Venrath, U. (2020): Mentalisierungsbasierte (MBT) und Übertragungsfokussierte Psychotherapie (TFP): Neue Ansätze für die Weiterentwicklung der Tiefenpsychologischen Psychotherapie (TP). *Psychodynamische Psychotherapie*, 19, 138–152.

Lombardi, R. (2017): *Body-Mind Dissociation in Psychoanalysis – Development after Bion*. New York: Routledge. Dtsch.

Lorenzer, A. (1973): *Sprachzerstörung und Rekonstruktion. Vorarbeiten zu einer Metatheorie der Psychoanalyse*. Frankfurt a. M.: Suhrkamp.

Malloch, S. & Trevarthen, C. (2009): *Communicative Musicality – Exploring the Basis of Human Companionship*. Oxford: Oxford University Press.

Masud Khan, M. (1977 [1963]): Das kumulative Trauma. In: Masud Khan, M. (Ed.): *Selbsterfahrung in der Therapie*. München: Kindler.

Ogden, T. O. (1995 [1989]): *Frühe Formen des Erlebens*. Trans. by H. Friessner & E.-M. Wolfram. Wien/New York: Springer.

Plassmann, R. (2011): *Selbstorganisation – Über Heilungsprozesse in der Psychotherapie*. Gießen: Psychosozial.

Plassmann, R. (2019): *Psychotherapie der Emotionen. Die Bedeutung von Emotionen für die Entstehung und Behandlung von Krankheiten*. Gießen: Psychosozial.

Ruettner, B., Goetzmann, L. & Siegel, A. (2015): "Der Sprung ins Imaginäre" – Zur behandlungstechnischen Verwendung psychosomatischer Körpersymptome. *Psyche – Z Psychoanal*, 69, 714–736.

Schreber, D. P. (1973 [1903]): *Denkwürdigkeiten eines Nervenkranken*. Frankfurt a. M.: Ullstein.

Schulz-Venrath, U. (2013): *Lehrbuch Mentalisieren – Psychotherapien wirksam gestalten*. Stuttgart: Klett-Cotta.

Schulz-Venrath, U. (2021): *Mentalisieren des Körpers*. Stuttgart: Klett-Cotta.

Stern, D. N. (2003 [1985]): *Die Lebenserfahrung des Säuglings*. Stuttgart: Klett-Cotta.

Stern, D. N. et al. (2002): Nicht-deutende Mechanismen in der psychoanalytischen Therapie. Das "Etwas-Mehr" als Deutung. *Psyche – Z Psychoanal*, 56, 974–1006.

Tronick, E. Z. (2007): *The Neurobehavioral and Social-Emotional Development of Infants and Children*. New York/London: Norton.

Tronick, E.Z. & Cohn, J. (1989): Infant mother face-to-face interaction: Age and gender differences in coordination and miscoordination. *Child Dev*, 59, 85–92.

Tsolas, V. & Anzieu-Premmereur, C. (2018): *A Psychoanalytic Exploration of the Body in Today's World*. London: Routledge.

Tustin, F. (2005): *Autistische Barrieren bei Neurotikern*. Trans. by K. O'Keeffe u. E. Vorspohl. Frankfurt a. M.: Brandes & Apsel.

van der Kolk, B. (2015): *Verkörperter Schrecken – Traumaspuren in Gehirn, Geist und Körper und wie man sie heilen kann*. Lichtenau/Westf.: Probst.

Volz-Boers, U. (2016): Resonanz im Körper des Analytikers. Das Konzept der sensorischintuitiven Haltung. In: Walz-Pawlita, S., Unruh, B. & Janta, B. (Eds.): *Körper-Sprachen*. Gießen: Psychosozial, 141–152.

Weinberg, K. M. & Tronick, E. Z. (1996): Infant affective reactions to the resumption of maternal interaction after the still-face. *Child Dev*, 67(3), 905–914.

Winnicott, D. W. (1989 [1969]): The mother-child experience of mutuality. In: Winnicott, C., Sherherd, R. & Davis M. (Eds.): *Psycho-Analytic Explorations*, 251–260.

Winnicott, D. W. (2018): Die Psychologie der Verrücktheit – Ein Beitrag der Psychoanalyse. *Psyche – Z Psychoanal*, 72(4), 254–266.

Chapter 7

"My Body Runs Alongside Me Like Something I Don't Need."

Bodily Sensations in the Development and Organization of Mental Structure

Ursula Volz-Boers

> Could it be that the development of mental structures requires specific actions that are not centered around meanings but around real interactions that generate new mental spaces, new programs? Though it may seem paradoxical, we are dealing here with divisive connections and connecting divisions. (Lempa, 2021, p. 36).

Introduction

Aristotle's understanding of corporeality was that the energy of the living body shapes the development of the soul. Accordingly, the soul represents the energy form of the body, and the body and soul act as aspects of a unified event. Storck (2016, p. 28) conveys this Aristotelian view when he writes that, "with reference to Aristotle, I support the concept that the vivacity of the body [...] is a constitutive, form-giving moment and the realization of the psyche's potentiality. [...] Mental life owes itself to a flowing-through of natural vibrancy."

In psychoanalytic work, we are increasingly challenged by patients who do not feel at home in their bodies. Rather, their body seems to them to lack such natural vibrancy. One of the possible causes of alienation from the body lies in the dissociation of body and soul. In this regard, Lombardi (2021 [2019]) writes that there is a difference in the dissonance of the two inner systems of body and psyche: dissonance with a traumatic origin and dissonance stemming from early life. Regarding the latter, he says:

> This disorder has its roots in the first months of life or even intrauterine, that is, in the premental period when the birth of the psyche, mediated by maternal reverie, "pushes the body into the background." (2021, p. 259)

Lombardi points out that people affected in this way pose great challenges to therapeutic communication, which "sometimes bring us to the very limits of our personal means and analytic methods. Omnipotent mental control is only

DOI: 10.4324/9781003370130-7

one of the possible configurations in which the psyche becomes an enemy of the body. When body and psyche enter a state of mutual alienation – as if belonging to different individuals – the disharmony may be even more pronounced, blocking the mental perception of inner sensations and feelings and paralyzing any chance of psychoanalytically working through the situation" (Lombardi, 2021, p. 259). This is what happened to my patient Julia, who provided the quote in the heading and whose story I report below.

Contemporary psychoanalysis is paying increasing attention to the bodily dimension (Anzieu, 1991 [1985]; Birkstedt-Breen, 2019; Hartung & Steinbrecher, 2018; Kobylinska-Dehe, 2019; Küchenhoff, 2012; Leikert, 2019; Lemma, 2018 [2015]; Leuzinger-Bohleber, 2009, Leuzinger-Bohleber et al., 2013; Lombardi, 2019; Plassmann, 2019; Scharff, 2010; Schultz-Venrath & Felsberger, 2016; Schultz-Venrath, 2021; Storck, 2016). Lemma writes that ego-structure and identity are rooted in bodily structures and an awareness of the body throughout life, and that Freud established the notion that the body-ego serves as a container and foundation for the sense of self:

The body always speaks. [...] It has a [...] pronounced presence in the analytic relationship, reflected in the analyst's somatic counter-transference, which captures the still unspoken history and gradually puts it into words." (Lemma, 2018 [2015], p. 27)

It is my experience as well that somatic countertransference is interconnected with ongoing processes in the therapist, referred to by such terms as presence, resonance, reverie, empathy, transformation from beta to alpha (Bion, 1990), implicit relational knowledge (Stern et al., 2012 [2010]), and embodiment (Leuzinger-Bohleber et al., 2013).

In addition to the body, contemporary psychoanalysis is also increasingly addressing intrauterine development – an infant's prenatal "programming" and its lifelong impact on human health and illness. Lombardi's reference above to the roots of dissociation in the premental and intrauterine period is part of a psychoanalytic developmental sequence that began with Rank (1924). Rank's description of his experiences and conclusions about prenatal and perinatal life and his implicit introduction into psychoanalysis of references to the feminine and maternal dimensions led to his estrangement with Freud. As is well known, Freud described his research predominantly in terms of his patients' experiences regarding the father relationship. According to Janus (2016, p. 242), Rank was more concerned with the "womb reality," "while Freud spoke only of the 'womb fantasies.' At the time, this disagreement could not be resolved, leading to Rank's departure from the close group of psychoanalysts." Ferenczi's (1982 [1929]) text on the subject of the unwelcome child proved to be seminal regarding the profound influence of the earliest rejections experienced by the child, conveyed in maternal and paternal sensations, fantasies, words, and behaviors.

In the 1990s, the Hungarian psychoanalysts Hidas and Raffai (2021 [2002]) developed a method of applying psychoanalysis as a means of early prevention of psychotic illness in childhood and adolescence. They called their method "Attachment Analysis: The Psychoanalytically Oriented Promotion of Prenatal Bonding Between Mother and Baby." Hidas and Raffai had observed that the mothers of psychotically ill adolescents had commonly suffered excessive stress during their pregnancies. The authors noted that, under these conditions, the maturation of the (proto)representations of the child's body-self and their differentiation from their maternal body-self representations may have been disrupted. The consequences of such intrauterine and perinatal experiences, they posited, could contribute postnatally to pathology in the experience of body-soul unity, self-object differentiation, and reality testing.

The "attachment analysis" method consists of emotionally accompanying the mother and, more recently, the father during pregnancy. The assumption that prenatal, perinatal, and early postnatal experiences remain physiologically bound in the sensomotor-affective system and can be reactivated throughout life in the form of spontaneously emerging bodily sensations and/or illnesses led Raffai to refer to this form of bodily sensation as the "language of intrauterine life" (2008). This reflected his view that the child's traumatic experiences in the womb are physiologically etched into bodily sensations and, because they are unrepresented, present themselves later, in postnatal life, as spontaneous bodily sensations.

These, in turn, can be processed in the therapeutic relationship through a mentalizing process, allowing them to further develop as feelings, images, fantasies, memories, thoughts, language, and meaning – and become linked with existing mental contents. I use the term mentalizing here in the sense of Fonagy (Fonagy et al., 2004 [2002]) as the ability to understand one's own affective states and the inner constitutions of other people as well as their interpersonal behavior. Schultz-Venrath adds bodily perception to the term: "Mentalizing is considered the ability to understand oneself and others regarding inner mental states closely connected to bodily perceptions" (2021, p. 14). Raffai (2008) applied the concept of mentalizing in transference particularly to those bodily sensations he considered as reactivating prenatal and perinatal experiences in the psychoanalytic process.

In the following, I use the example of the 32-year-old Julia to present my psychoanalytic concept of "working with bodily sensations from a sensory-intuitive stance" within the context of countertransference, transference, and resistance. Julia was consumed by a desperate postnatal condition when she sought help with her 6-week-old daughter, Mina. After describing the initial situation with Julia and Mina, I introduce the concepts of authors who support my interventions and my reflections, outline my method for working with bodily sensations, and describe treatment sessions that illustrate them. The initial interviews led to my offering Mina and Julia baby therapy and extended to individual psychoanalytic therapy with Julia. In both settings, baby therapy and analytic psychotherapy, I worked with "touch," conveyed with my presence, resonance, empathy, voice, and words, whereas I did not work with tactile touch.

The Child Who Could Not Be Taken from the Mother's Body

Julia made an appointment by phone because her gynecologist had repeatedly advised her to do so. She had to come together with her child, she said, because her daughter could not be removed from her side without crying unbearably and inconsolably. When the very slim and petite Julia came to my consultation with the sleeping Mina in her arms, she was in bad shape: exhausted, pale, emaciated, with a fearful, desperate look on her face. She triggered in me the feeling of wanting to put my arms around her in a silent hug to protect and strengthen her. As if unconsciously resisting the vibrations from my countertransference, Julia began by saying,

> I only came here because of Mina. My gynecologist urgently advised me to clear things up, to check whether everything is all right with Mina. I don't believe in psychotherapy, and I don't believe in talking about the past. I think people behave the way they are, which has nothing to do with their family or their past. I'm not interested in any nonsense from the past. The only thing is: Even though I have my baby in my arms all the time and am so close to her, I can't understand what she wants. I basically don't understand Mina. I'm a perfectionist and doing my best, but apparently that's not enough for her. I just can't be a good mother. I've hardly had anything to eat or drink for three days. The breast infection is killing me when I breastfeed. At night I sleep with Mina right on top of my body. I can only sleep from maybe 2 to 4 in the morning for fear that something bad might happen if I take care of myself. This fear started early in pregnancy.

I initially listened to Julia's distress and fears in silent attention, feeling wary of asking for content too early, before Julia, Mina, and I had developed an extended bond of incipient safety and trust. I believed Julia sensed the compassion in my voice when I told her, "I find what you are confiding in me very important and sad. You are bravely dealing with a difficult situation."

Julia shrugged her shoulders. Mina continued to sleep motionlessly in her mother's arms, her little head resting on Julia's left shoulder. Mina looked as if she hadn't quite arrived in the outside world yet. It occurred to me that perhaps she had indeed not yet been born spiritually, or that she was putting her liveliness at her mother's service. Julia described how Mina slept practically 24 hours a day, did not open her eyes when nursing or her diapers were being changed; she did not respond to being spoken to by her parents or her 3-year-old brother. "Yet, Mina was a dream child for my husband and me. She also screams terribly when he tries to pick her up. Thankfully, he takes care of our son." I learned that the son, too, had screamed throughout his first year of life. During the pregnancy with him, Julia had suffered from a fear that something bad might happen, though it was weaker than with Mina. Julia gave birth to the son spontaneously, whereas with Mina she had insisted on having a C-section. "Today, I'm much more desperate than I was in the early days with my son."

In another preliminary interview, I learned of Julia's close relationship with her identical twin sister and the comfort she received from her marriage to her husband of the same age – except for her chronic fear of his abandoning her should she become a nuisance or show him that she not only liked him but loved him. I could sense her fear of also not being wanted or considered a nuisance in the therapeutic relationship and of being abandoned as soon as the therapist became important to her. After completing her studies and starting a family, she had worked part-time as a manager. She confided in me that her nonstop activity served to avoid feelings and prove her usefulness. She could not be alone, could not stand silence or darkness.

Her parents were 22 years old when her mother unintentionally became pregnant, and even in the the delivery room, she did not know that she was going to have twins. When the twin sister was born first, the parents were disappointed in "having to have" Julia as a second child. Initially, they had a name for the twin sister but not for Julia, so she remained nameless for several days. Julia's maternal grandmother, with whom Julia had a good relationship as long as she did everything the grandmother dictated, said repeatedly: "Nobody was happy to see you arrive. I didn't want your mother as a second child after my first daughter either."

At the time of our initial interviews, Julia's mother was suffering from multiple sclerosis and a recurrence of ovarian cancer. Regarding her relationship with her mother, Julia said,

> To this day, my mother keeps telling me that I am difficult, complicated, that I drive her crazy, that I am to blame for her illness, and that I should leave her alone with my questions. Her frequent phrase was, "Nobody cares about what you're asking." She made a fool of me. Since I was a child, I constantly tried not to be difficult, to behave in such a way that I didn't disturb anyone, didn't burden anyone, didn't complicate anything, didn't need anything. I am constantly trying to grasp what other people expect of me.

She described her father as generally calmer, with no opinion of his own besides her mother's. He failed to protect Julia when the mother hit her. He also beat Julia, though less frequently. Her other sister, 3 years younger, whom Julia frequently had to take care of at her parents' behest during childhood and adolescence, suffered from "schizophrenia." The parents separated when Julia was 18. Throughout all of these conversations during our therapy sessions, the baby continued to lie immobile on Julia's shoulder. When I said, "It hurts me to think of what you have suffered. I care about your thoughts and your questions," she responded with, "Well, I don't care."

In the third preliminary interview, Julia confided in me that she had been preoccupied throughout the entire pregnancy with Mina with the agonizing thought that the baby might die. She had been able to trust the ultrasound image of the living child only for a short time and had thereafter hardly felt any movements in her body, if at all. During the last month of pregnancy, the thought of her child dying became unbearable, which is why she asked for a Cesarean section on her due date, hoping that her fear of a dead child would disappear the moment she could "see her living child, take care of it, and assume control over it with all her efforts."

When Julia spoke of controlling the baby, I guessed that "control" meant something positive to her and provided stability. She added that she had experienced a brief moment of happiness at the sight of Mina after the C-section. But that quickly faded against the haunting notion that Mina might die after all.

During this narrative, Mina began to cry more and more. Julia mentioned that she had breastfed Mina shortly before our appointment and was sure she was not crying from hunger. Mina had cried louder and louder since the mother mentioned her thoughts of the child's death. I decided to use a baby-therapeutic intervention (after Terry, 2008–2012), which I present below.

No Body, No Sensations – Reflections on Julia's Suffering

My understanding of Julia's experience of rejection and loneliness gradually began to take shape. I was struck by the extent to which she failed to recognize her despair, hatred, and longing as the result of withheld love and experienced rejection, instead projecting them into her body or dissociating herself completely from the experiences. Several questions arose in me: Had Julia been allowed to accept and shape the life she had received from her mother and father against her mother's will? Did she recognize herself in her present existence, where she had succeeded in many things? Or did she have to punish herself with self-hatred for not having died in her mother's womb or at birth – as she imagined her mother had wished all along? Did Julia connect with her mother's fantasized death wish through imitation (Gaddini, 2015)? Was she projecting it onto her own daughter, whose imminent death she had expected? Her inner world seemed to be missing the experience of unmitigated joy about herself and acceptance. Would Julia have been less tormented by fears of her child's death – and, I assume, her fear of her own death – if she had been sheltered by and understood by her mother's dreamy sense of foreboding (Beland, 2020)?

Beland (2020) writes of the nameless fear of persons whose fear of life is not acknowledged at the beginning and fails to be transformed into a trust in shared life. If Julia had experienced being welcomed, would she then perhaps not have had to always "earn" her place in life via nonstop activity? If she hadn't had to constantly assess what others – supposedly – were expecting of her and adjust her behavior correspondingly using constant control to avoid difficulties, conflicts, rejection, devaluation, and a fear of unpleasant feelings? She later once said,

> I don't want to feel anything unpleasant. I always feel misunderstood. I don't even want to have a body. My body runs alongside me like something I don't really need. I can turn it on and off like a lamp. I don't feel it, so I can control it. I can go for three days without eating. But the feeling of being hungry or thirsty is unbearable for me. I don't want to be dependent on a feeling.

Julia's statement that her body was a "thing" that "runs alongside" her through life triggered both wonderment and concern in me because of the expressed remoteness from her body and the depersonalization. At the same time, because of the depth of her suffering and her existing healthy ego, I also felt hope: As her escort, her body had at least remained mobile and not rigid. Furthermore, I could foresee the gap between the overemphasis of her controlling thinking and her denial of bodily sensations giving way to new mental spaces during our work, namely, if a psychoanalytic interaction were to succeed that included the bodily sensations of the patient *and* the psychoanalyst.

Application of Theory When Dealing with Corporeality

As a theoretical background for working with the body in psychoanalysis, I use the concepts of presence (Gumbrecht, 2004, 2012; Schmidt, 2014; Stern, 2014 [2004]; Wolf et al., 2018), resonance (Schore, 2009), embodiment (Leuzinger-Bohleber et al., 2013), autistic-touching position (Ogden, 1995 [1989]), and autonomous body memory (Leikert, 2019; see also Volz-Boers, 2016). Gumbrecht, Schmidt, Wolf, and colleagues emphasize body-related emotional encounters that spontaneously emerge in fleeting moments of feeling present. Ogden (1995 [1989]) describes the autistic-touching approach as a mode of experiential formation in which sensory input – particularly of the skin surface – and the experience of rhythm form a budding sense of self. He writes:

> The experience of the "self" [...] is derived from bodily needs that only gradually become ego needs, just as a psychology gradually emerges from the imaginative elaboration of a bodily experience (in the mother-infant relationship). (Winnicott cited after Ogden, 1995 [1989], p. 33).

That sounds like a blueprint for the psychoanalyst's dealing with patients like Julia, who convey an absence of sufficient experiences of resonance, fantasy, and imaginative involvement with their bodily needs and the transition thereof into psychological content in their early parental relationship. Leikert (2019, p. 27), in his image of "encapsulated body engrams," describes somatic configurations, that is, patterns of innervation, that fail to make contact in both directions:

> They have lost contact with the reasons behind the phenomena and can no longer connect to the spontaneous process of imagination, i.e., the transformation of a bodily sensation into an expressive gestalt, whether in dreams or as a fantasy (ibid.).

Applying a Sensory-Intuitive Approach to Working with Bodily Sensations

When working with unrepresented or insufficiently represented corporeal phenomena, using a sensory-intuitive approach seems to me to be helpful. The first component of the term – "sensory" –denotes a perception that focuses on the sensation of spontaneously occurring, sensually felt bodily feelings, which usually leads to resonance in the analyst's body as well (Volz-Boers, 2016). "Intuitive," in turn, means a foreboding grasp of the "capacity for imaginative perception of unconscious messages [...] that elude logical-denotative thinking [...]" (Warsitz, 2014, p. 857). Furthermore,

> The dream-like ability of a mother to foresee or interpret the child's unadapted signals, on which the child elementally depends if they want to make sense of them, does not originate from a cognitive process of perception but from an intuitive ability more akin to poetic or esthetic functions (ibid.).

On the Theoretical Understanding of Bodily Sensations

I use the term "bodily sensation" to address sensory stimuli that emerge spontaneously. These include sensations from the surface of the skin (surface sensibility, exteroception), from the organs (interoception), and from sensations of posture and movement in space as well as other information from inside the body, which comprise part of depth sensibility and bodily sensation in the form of proprioception. Spontaneous bodily sensations belong to experiences that are mentally unrepresented or insufficiently represented. They are presymbolic and extraverbal and belong to the implicit memory contents.

Stern et al. (2012 [2010]) pointed out that, because of modern memory research, we can now distinguish two domains of therapeutic change in psychoanalysis: the explicit (or declarative) and the implicit (or procedural). Processes that occur in the explicit, declarative realm are conscious or almost conscious; they are symbolized and thus linguistically graspable: Contents of the repressed, dynamic unconscious are assigned to this declarative realm. On the explicit level lie free association, proportionate attention, and semantic interpretations, which alter the patient's intrapsychic understanding and contribute to their psychic reorganization.

On the other hand, the ability to sense and name bodily sensations as part of the therapeutic interaction means working with implicit, procedural memory content. These experiences, because they are not yet represented or symbolized, are not accessible through thoughts and words, that is, through free association. According to Stern, they can be reorganized only in the presence of new experiences in relational moments.

In my experience, procedural memory contents become attainable and changeable by perceiving bodily sensations during the psychoanalytic treatment process. This aspect complements Stern's descriptions cited above (Volz-Boers, 2016).

What conditions lead to the representation and development of the symbolic failing to be achieved or going missing altogether? If we assume the reactivation of prenatal, perinatal, and early postnatal experiences, we can discover patterns of experiential processing in the therapeutic relationship in which experience remains physiologically bound to bodily sensations – on the sensomotoric-affective level of organization of experience.

Accordingly, we understand Mina's behavior such that, during development, the child failed to experience sufficient incipient representations or protorepresentations of the boundaries of its body-self and was thus unable to detach itself after birth, even temporarily, from contact with the mother's body. According to current knowledge, we may assume that reduced or missing representation is a sign not only of a very early developmental stage but can also result from deprivational relationship experiences and attachment deficits. Furthermore, psychological traumatization hinders the formation of representations and/or is accompanied by the destruction of already-developed representations (Volz-Boers, 1999).

The Methodology of Working with Bodily Sensations

When working with bodily sensations, the ability to allow for not-knowing and uncertainty plays an important role. In this regard, Fenichel writes: "One perceives the other by experiencing their qualities through one's own bodily sensations" (Fenichel quoted after Ogden, 1995 [1989], p. 77). In working with the bodily sensations of patients, the psychoanalyst attunes their own bodily sensations in the act of feeling and analyzing, which means an additional effort and challenge in the therapeutic process. Methodologically speaking, working with bodily sensations demands directing one's empathic attention to bodily sensations and associations, in addition to using free association regarding thoughts and feelings and equal attention.

This process takes place within the matrix of countertransference, transference, and resistance, in an empathic relational setting that conveys safety and is resonant to bodily sensations. Such interventions related to bodily sensations run in phases and are offered *before* working with feelings, thoughts, and interpretations. Thus, the goal is to foster the ability to *sense* and *feel* before thinking kicks in. In the binary interplay of seeking sensations and thinking representations, perceptual awareness is temporarily directed more toward the sensory experience of both patient and analyst than toward interpretive hermeneutics.

If the patient succeeds in becoming increasingly involved with visualizing bodily sensations, they can gradually transform them into feelings, images, fantasies, thoughts, and words in a mentalizing work process. Depending on the situation, the occasional follow-up offer of a narrative can support the patient's search for meaning and sense. But a narrative is often unnecessary because the patient grasps the meaning of their bodily sensations themselves once they have developed into feelings, images, memories, and language. Working with them proceeds alternately in the presence of both explicit and implicit memory contents.

The Technique of Working with Bodily Sensations

In the practical work with bodily sensations, in addition to applying free association, it is a matter of attuning oneself to the free-flowing bodily sensations. To reach the level of bodily associations, the analyst should wisely extend the basic rule of attending to bodily sensations: Patients are offered the chance to talk about anything that comes to mind, whether thoughts, memories, imaginations, or feelings they have never talked about before. And they are asked to articulate *what* and *how* they feel *in their bodies*. For example, if the patient talks about some bodily discomfort or pain, these are picked up in subsequent questions. This connects the patient's sensations to their bodily experience. For example, if the patient speaks of pain in the chest, then, in my experience, the analyst can best support the discovery process by directing their sensibility to their own body area the patient is concerned about.

The following questions – tactfully timed and selectively posed – are usually helpful:

- Are you feeling your anxiety (anger, loneliness, lostness, etc.) in your body right now?
- Where do you perceive the pain in your body?
- Can you let yourself be guided further by your body signal?
- Can you go into your bodily sensation?

- Can you follow your bodily sensation?
- Can you become one with your bodily sensation?

Such questions prepare you to ask: "What does it mean?" I encourage letting the bodily sensations rule, staying with them for a few minutes, feeling whether further bodily sensations become noticeable, and then – often only after longer work – gradually and patiently perceiving whether and how these bodily sensations develop and transform into emotions, images, and words.

How the Analyst Deals with Their Own Bodily Sensations

This work requires sensitization of the psychoanalyst's ability to perceive, not the least their own bodily sensations, which can take place most effectively as part of a psychoanalytic self-experience that includes the bodily dimension of experience. Evaluating one's own coenesthetic sensations is an important analytic instrument when working with the sensomotoric-affective functional parts of the ego – as it is in dealing with the intense archaic rage of patients. Using one's own body as a resonance space for the sensomotoric elements of the patient's transference has the effect of dealing with the patient's body without ever touching it. Using questions to focus on the deepened sensing of the patient's emerging bodily sensations (see below) silently directs questions toward the analyst:

- How do I feel during this?
- How do I perceive what I am sensing, what is conveyed to me in resonance, fantasy, intuition, imagination, and embodied countertransference?
- Do I trust the fantasies that resonate in me?
- How do I process what I am sensing, perceiving, and discovering in accordance with psychoanalytic methodology?

Both the patient and the analyst may experience anxiety while working with bodily sensations as well as intense experiences of being at the mercy of the other – of powerlessness, helplessness, and even fear of annihilation. These fears may be accompanied by the experience of falling into a chasm or black hole or of floating endlessly in infinite space. There may be the feeling that the boundaries of one's own body or the internal surfaces of the body are dissolving, the perception of leaking out, disintegrating, or becoming rigid. If an analyst feels sufficiently confident in experiencing and dealing with their own resonance toward protosensory and protoemotional constitutions, patients may then increasingly dare to move toward allowing them to emerge in the analytic relationship – by employing the ego strength they have gathered during the work with the bodily sensations.

The Baby-Therapeutic Experience with Mina and Julia

As Julia spoke more extensively of her intolerable fears, to the point of her having been convinced that the child inside her was dying, Mina cried louder and louder, heartbreakingly. Through the crying, Julia said, "Since the C-section, I am consumed with the additional, lingering guilt of having damaged Mina because of my desire to have her delivered surgically. Is that why she doesn't want to leave my side? I can't stand it when she cries; it makes me want to cry with her."

I saw the tears in Julia's eyes and asked her, "Can you accept and tolerate Mina's crying together with me? Show her through comforting sounds and little words that you are there for her. By crying, Mina can share her pain, perhaps cry it out, and let go of it. You and I can take it in. I will support you in this. In doing so, Mina can feel that she is not alone but comforted. If you feel you can't take Mina's crying anymore, show it to me. You mustn't overwhelm yourself. And it mustn't become too much for Mina. If you feel that's happening, you can comfort Mina with your breast or a pacifier as usual – as you see fit." Mina continued to cry, loudly and touchingly. Julia replied that she would try with me to accept and tolerate Mina's crying. I still asked Julia if I could talk to Mina. The mother nodded in agreement.

I got up and stood behind Julia's chair, so I could see Mina's face on her mother's shoulder. (In this case, my moving around the room had only the practical goal of being able to see the baby's face. I did not apply any scenic work with my steps toward the child and mother.) Then I asked Mina if I could say something to her. She opened her eyes and looked at me. While I began to speak the following in a soft, calm, and quiet voice, Mina stopped crying and continued to look at me, unblinkingly:

> Mina, your Mama and your Papa are happy that you are alive. Now I'll say something sad: When you were in Mama's womb, Mama was afraid that you might die. This fear your Mama had comes from her life story. But it's not your story. When you sleep on Mama's tummy, you show her that you are alive. But you don't have to, and in fact you can't help your Mama that way. If Mama wants to, together she and I can try to take care of her – until she gets better. You may separate your body from your Mama's body whenever you want, so that you can continue to discover life and the world in your own way.

At this point, Mina's eyes fell shut. She fell asleep. I was moved, grateful, and amazed. Mina's reaction is not sufficiently explainable to me, according to what I now know.

Julia was amazed. As she gently placed Mina in the carrier, the child continued to sleep. Julia asked for another appointment, which she attended without her child. She reported that Mina had slept for another 3 hours at home after the session – alone in her crib near her parents. Since then, Mina seemed more awake, looking at her parents, smiling, closely observing her surroundings, and letting her father take her in his arms. At night, Mina slept in her own bed. When I said, "Mina continued her psychic birth," Julia asked, "What did you do?" I answered more or less as follows:

> You were there, you saw and heard everything. Above all, I saw and heard what you did: You allowed me to talk to the screaming Mina. I think Mina heard and perceived that. Then, you gave Mina's crying space – for a long time. You were there for Mina while she cried. She was able to accept something, which incited change. It's as if Mina began to be more in her own body instead of turning her body to that of her mother for reassurance. As a result, she could sleep apart from you, while still being deeply connected to you: She now looks at you and smiles with you. Despite everything that is incomprehensible in this sequence of events, perhaps this one thing we can understand: You had the strength to accept Mina's pain, longing, despair, and anger in her crying. Maybe Mina felt she no longer had to show her mother that she was alive by continually being near her. You confided in me that your mother felt overwhelmed by you as the second twin child. Like Mina, and like your mother, you are the second child. Maybe you didn't know whether you were allowed to live or whether it would have been better if you were dead so that your mother could be better off. This idea may have led to your conviction, which then morphed into the agonizing thought of Mina's death during your second pregnancy. Let us try to work on reconnecting the two sides of your conflict: being allowed to live and enjoy the life your parents gave you in your own way, and your deep fear that if you do embrace and create life, your parents will be punished with death.

"Oh," Julia responded, "now I understand my suicidal impulses. During puberty, I had anorexia and thought of eating rat poison. Your conjectures have made a light come on in my head. But I don't feel anything. I'm just afraid Mina will die while I take care of myself or sleep."

In response to my offer that she and I could together look closely at her anxiety, thought patterns, and bodily feelings, she said, "Mina is doing better since I was here with her. That gives me hope. I want to change my obsessive thinking, seem less weird and complicated to others, and find a new order in my mind."

Understanding and Shaping the Psychoanalytic Situation with Julia

I offered Julia seated psychotherapy for the first year for 1 hour per week. To me, 1 hour a week seemed appropriate to allow for the gradual development of rapprochement in the therapeutic relationship. As Julia gained more confidence and security in her contact with me (and I with her), we continued with 3 hours per week, mostly recumbent. It was my recommendation that she lie on the couch so that she could better tune into her bodily sensations without interference.

I began to work more frequently with the methodology described earlier. Julia's initial reaction to the offer of increased frequency confirmed her increased confidence in the therapeutic relationship: "Do you want to work with me more so you can get rid of me faster?" I told her that, by asking this question, she was showing courage that would not have been possible a few months ago. Now, she said, she could negotiate her mistrust and rage over her perceived rejection by her mother and father with me. Afterward, she said, "It's not like I'm doing this on purpose, coming up with this. But I also feel a bit of joy that you're taking even more time for me, and I like coming three times a week despite my fear that our work will become so important to me that I'll become dependent."

The patient's mental structure included healthy and viable areas in which she could love and work, embrace her marriage, and care for her children, which she managed well enough with her husband: Their partnership and the children thrived. Her mental organization, which included the symbolized area of experience processing that had become unconscious through defense mechanisms, was expressed in her compulsively controlling and distrustful parts as well as her narcissistic patterns in dealing with herself and others. They were assigned to the *explicit* memory contents.

Further, in her presymbolic and subsymbolic experiences, that is, in her *implicit* memory contents, lay a dissociation between body and psyche, which resulted in her anorexia (165 cm, 40 kg). Her lack of body self-coherence and her insecure maternal attachment, among other things, seemed to have prevented Julia from using her aggressive power of differentiation to delineate the internal image of her life design from the internal image of her mother's life design for her. Julia dissociated her impulses toward annihilation and matricidal revenge, which translated into her fears about Mina's dying. For a long time, they seemed inaccessibly enclosed, recalling Leikert's (2019) concept of "encapsulated body engrams."

I learned that Julia found her inner world threatening in ways she could not understand or regulate, which caused her tremendous anxiety. At night, she would lie awake for hours, checking the darkness with her eyes open, fearing she would vanish into thin air in the darkness if she closed her eyes. She could not be alone in the apartment; she could not eat at her mother's and grandmother's house because she could not free herself from the thought that both of them had poisoned her food – but not the food of her husband and children. Only after 3 years of therapy did she confide in me about the neurodermatitis on her scalp (which I hadn't noticed). She also dealt with it according to her tried and true motto: "What I don't notice doesn't exist."

During this time, she first mentioned that her mother had beaten her every morning during her elementary school years. She hadn't understood why. At some point, the mother said she hit Julia as a precaution to prevent her from asking annoying questions or acting "difficult." I experienced her telling me these terrible stories as a vote of confidence in our relationship. Until then, Julia had withheld such information to prevent me from thinking how right her mother had been in seeing Julia as a bad person. She said: "If someone knows that I was beaten, it's proof that not just one person thinks I deserve to be beaten."

I replied, "I think – and indeed am completely convinced – that you did not deserve her beatings. At the same time, I experience it as progress that you are communicating your concern that I *might* think the same way as your mother." She responded, "I don't want to shift any experiences with my mother onto you. That would be unfair." "Let it happen," I said. "It's part of our work to allow what has been beaten down in you to grow back in our relationship. I believe that a new inner life can emerge if we can give space to and thus detoxify the experiences and feelings concerning your mother who rejected and beat you."

Julia responded, "I don't know how to do that."

When, in the third year of analysis, she mentioned that the fear of Mina's dying was no longer present, I told her that, from this example, she was experiencing how new spaces with more trust could emerge in her. Julia's outward appearance changed over the first 2 years of therapy compared to the beginning: She began to wear more colored clothes that looked good on her. A slight weight gain (she now weighed 46 kg) made her pretty face appear softer.

I would now like to present some excerpts from the path to these incipient and positive changes using a dream of hers and excerpts from the treatment sessions.

A Dream

Julia told me this dream during the second year of treatment:

> I am in another country with my twin sister. We are being followed by people who all look the same, like multiples or clones, but they are all the same person. We are swimming in a circle in a swimming pool. The persons do not come into the water but wait on the side. If you go out of the water, they want to kill you. We are looking for a way out of the water but can't get out because they would have recognized us by our wet clothes. Then someone is swimming behind me in the water, he wants to grab me, and I say to him, "If you kill me, I'll reveal your secret." After that, the person takes the outstretched hand away from me, swims to shore, and says to the others there she has not found us. Then I woke up.

Asked about her ideas about the dream, Julia said, "What ideas? It's not like I chose the dream. What do you mean by 'ideas'? Do you mean I'm dramatizing?"

"I'm not thinking you're dramatizing, but I'm wondering what feelings and bodily sensations you had in the dream."

"In the dream, I felt fear and despair. But not now. I never go into swimming pools, and I never go into bathtubs. Just lying around there, that's awful. My mom used to pull the plug out of the tub when we were still in it. I was afraid I'd be sucked down the drain. My mom always showered us off with cold water so we wouldn't complain about the cold. I was glad when I got through it. I think I was probably 2 years old. I don't know if you can remember things that early. I do remember it being uncomfortable."

"You're starting to trust your memories and the feelings that go with them more. In the dream, you know about a secret."

"That the person was going to kill me, that was the secret. I barely escaped with my life – I think that's good. But that the person lied to others? I don't think lying is good. It's important to me that there's no lying going on."

I was amazed at the potential and "knowledge" of her dream-self. But also about how far the knowledge of her dream consciousness still was from the knowledge of her waking consciousness. For a long time, she warded off the cautious hints in the dream to accept her own aggressive power to come out of the water alive by simply not understanding. She seemed to distance herself from perceiving her own killing impulses. This dream accompanied the further process.

Working with Bodily Sensations During Treatment Sessions

Once, when I noticed her rapid breathing, I counted the number of breaths: 32 a minute. I was looking for a way to determine whether she was excited or scared at that moment and asked her about it.

Julia said, "I look forward to the time here. But when I'm here, I don't know what to say at the outset without being difficult and complicated."

"I believe that what is difficult and complicated is human. If it gets the necessary space, attention, and understanding between us, then it can change. May I share an observation with you without criticizing you or making you take a cold shower here?"

"Yes."

"Normally, we take about 16 breaths a minute. In doing so, we exhale longer than we inhale. However, I've noticed that you breathe faster and exhale shorter. That's why I asked you earlier if you were excited or scared."

"It's not like I'm doing this on purpose. I've never thought about my breathing before."

"Then perhaps this is a good opportunity to do so. Your rapid breathing may reflect your uncertainty at the beginning of the hour." I silently think about her uncertainty at the beginning of life. "At the same time, your way of breathing may have become habitual and automated. Your brain would probably adopt a calmer breathing rhythm if you gave it the impetus to do so – like when we lose the beat while dancing and have to give ourselves a nudge to get back in rhythm."

She answered, obligingly, "I will try to pay better attention to that."

In the following account, I select a few therapy situations in which Julia got in touch with her heartbeat, with her windpipe, with the black void inside her. And I add a session in which we laughed heartily for the first time. After that, she spoke for the first time about her scalp and emerging sadness.

Julia became increasingly familiar with working with spontaneously occurring bodily sensations. But it took much time and patience until she could engage more with what she was sensing, feeling, and perceiving. She asked, "How do I know that my bodily sensations, like the tightness in my throat, the pressure in my head, or my heart palpitations, are real? Maybe I'm just imagining them?"

My explanation that spontaneously arising bodily sensations are not subject to our conscious will did little to convince her. More compelling were her experiences in which the bodily sensation changed or developed into feelings, words, an enhanced sense of understanding – and sometimes new behavior. It amazed her that, here and there, she was experiencing relief in the process, even though she had not exerted herself as much as usual.

The Heart Rhythm Is Experienced as Part of the Self

Julia talked about how she had not wanted to feel her heartbeat: It was too fast, made her restless, felt foreign to her, and she did not know whether it was coming from the outside or the inside. When she lay awake at night, she could not distinguish whether the "rhythmic sound" was coming from her, her husband next to her, or her pillow. She left the window wide open at night so that the sounds from the street would override the unpleasant sounds in her room or body. When I asked her whether she could feel her heartbeat in her body right now, 3 minutes of silence followed. I connected myself with my own heart and waited.

Julia finally spoke: "I have a hollow feeling in the middle of my chest. Around that pit, I feel my heartbeat, rising up to my throat and head. My throat feels tight. And in the tightness, I can feel the heartbeat most clearly." After another silence of about 3 minutes, she continued: "The pit is now subsiding. Now I feel my heart rhythm more at the front of my chest. The tightness in the throat is subsiding. With the heart rhythm comes a lighter feeling spreading upward from the chest." I was touched that she had stayed calm and concentrated after sensing her heart rhythm and said, "By sensing and describing your heartbeat in the last few minutes, you have found and maintained a connection to your heart rhythm."

"So far, only my heartbeat has bothered me. I wanted it to go away. Beyond that, I've never dealt with it before."

She began the next lesson this way: "Yesterday, I was able to accept something, to take possession of something: my heartbeat. I briefly felt that it belonged to me, that it was mine. I felt relief. Otherwise, my heart rhythm scared me. It helped that you said it was *my* heart rhythm. That it belonged *to me*; it gave the heartbeat a shape. Then I realized, wow, it must be coming from me, it's *my* heartbeat. Yesterday, when you said that I was in touch with my heartbeat, I thought, 'That's right. It wasn't like that before.'"

To which I responded: "By feeling a connection with your heart rhythm, you are experiencing one of your inner sources of strength. That can also give you a kind of independence, despite all human dependency and fear of dependency."

Her response of "Yes, thank you" sounded heartfelt.

I thought of how, as a twin in the womb, she had also heard her sister's heartbeat, which may have been like her own in rhythm – in addition to her mother's slower heartbeat. Could hearing three heart rhythms have perhaps made it more difficult for her to feel and accept her own heart rhythm as something belonging to her? When I shared this question with her, she responded briskly, "Every time you explain something like that to me, the unpleasant feelings in me subside."

Discovering the Trachea

During the COVID lockdown, I saw Julia only on a screen, sitting in her living room on her sofa, surrounded by colorful pillows. The greater closeness of her face under these circumstances – compared to the situation in the consulting room – triggered tender, motherly feelings in me several times.

She began one particular session while sitting: "I orient myself toward what I hear and see, so I have something to do, which distracts me from feeling anything." Julia's orientation toward the visible and the audible, as something controllable she could use to resist feeling, cost me much strength and patience. I knew that directly addressing such resistance was not (yet) a helpful tactic; my attempts to do so in the past had triggered tears and withdrawal – as well as again and again the statement: "I'm not doing this on purpose."

During this session, I responded to Julia's communication pattern with lethargy and the impulse to slump off to sleep. At the same time, I wanted to make space for resisting her feelings. It occurred to me that, in my embodied countertransference, I would also perceive her tiredness, despite her constant efforts not to be tired. Until then, she had repeatedly told me that she did not experience fatigue but was always in action and rarely wound down. She would sleep from about 1 to 2.30 a.m. and then again from 5 to 6 a.m. At 6 a.m., she would get up. On the screen, I could see that she was lying on her living room sofa, her eyes closed. "When I close my eyes, I don't feel any limits."

To my response, "I want to understand what you mean by limits," she said, "When my eyes are closed, I can tell exactly where my head ends and the pillow begins. Besides my head, though, everything else – the rest of my body – feels like water vapor or something."

"Can you go into the water vapor, follow it?"

"I guess I can try. But water vapor is not quite the right word. It's more like the body is lost, all mushy. I can't feel my body. My head is like a ball; my body is like a piece of cloth."

This sparked an image – like in a dream – I wanted to share with her so that she could understand that she was triggering something in another person that could have meaning: "If, in addition to your hearing and seeing what you alluded to earlier, you also engage with that sensation, you feel like a ball. This strikes me as an image drawn from earliest life. The human body starts out as a sphere surrounded by water and egg skins. Maybe egg skins could act like a piece of cloth?"

Seeming stimulated by this thought, she said, "How good that I talked about it. At first, I didn't want to say anything because it seemed so complicated and stupid. The fact that you can see something meaningful in it makes me feel more confident."

At the beginning of the following session, she said, "I'm beginning to understand the importance of sensations. Until now, I was convinced I could learn almost anything if I just decided to and tried hard enough. In school, I memorized everything, could reproduce it, got good grades, but I didn't really understand what I had memorized. For example, I memorized everything about nonviolence and thought what I learned with my head I could apply in life. Lately, I've realized that just learning isn't enough."

"How do you feel such things?"

"Well, yesterday, I first thought that if I say something, it will come out complicated, so I'd better not say anything. Then I did say something, and you and I understood something."

"I think you are becoming more confident in our relationship and more courageous in and with yourself."

"Something is changing in my interaction with my kids, too. My son showed me a bruise on his foot that hurt. For the first time, I didn't say what I usually say: 'Oh, stop whining. Don't act like that, don't look at it, and it won't hurt.' Instead, I put ointment on the sore spot and looked with him for shoes that wouldn't hurt."

"You've become more compassionate in your interactions with your son. A change is going on in your mothering behavior. It's as if you are creating a new space to be a mother. And your motherliness differs from that of your mother."

She smiled, lay down on the sofa, and began, "The top part of my head, behind my eyes, and the back part of my head feel heavy right now, heavier than the rest of the head. I feel like there's a boulder in my head."

"Can you follow the sensation in your head?"

"My face, shoulders, and arms feel cold, my neck feels warm. My eyes are also warm. I want to follow the warmth because it occupies more space in my neck and eyes than the cold. My whole face feels warm, all the way up to my neck. Below my neck is a hollow feeling."

"Would you like to go into the hollow?"

"It goes all the way under the breastbone. Like a hollow line. As though there's something outside of that hollow, as though the hollow line is an airless space."

"How do you feel about this airless line?"

"Neutral."

Listening to her, I felt a resonance in my windpipe. When she nodded her agreement to my question about whether I could say something to her about the hollow line, I offered this: "It seems to me that this hollow line might reflect your trachea – your windpipe."

"That's amazing! I didn't even know where the trachea was. Now I can feel it. I'm glad that I can. It's like I'm being gifted a trachea. I couldn't feel it before. At least by just trying."

A Little Brightness in the Black Darkness

At the beginning of one of the next sessions, Julia told about an encounter she had with her mother the previous weekend. "She has such a fixed stare. Since childhood I've had a hard time when she stares at me like that but doesn't look at me when I tell her something." Julia lay down and said, "When I close my eyes, I feel a lot of darkness and emptiness – it scares me. Of course, 'a lot' and 'emptiness' are a contradiction. The darkness spreads out, immediately suffocating everything else. I feel like I'm in shock."

I felt a tightness in my own throat and said, "Can you go further into the darkness? I'm right here with you."

"That's reassuring. At first, it feels like I'm alone. Then my head and upper body feel like they're dissolving, like there's no boundary. It's different only in the lower part of the neck and the upper part of my chest. I feel pressure. It's a little tight." After being silent for 2–3 minutes, she continues, speaking slowly, "It feels like the tightness is dark, all black, like very black air. It feels like this blackness is dissolving, melting, flowing. The blackness is heavy and cold. But there's a point below the neck that doesn't dissolve. It is separated from the blackness. And it's warmer. It feels lighter."

"Can you follow the lighter and warmer parts, too?"

"It's getting lighter. And has a little more shape to it. It's round."

I was impressed that she could allow both: The dark coldness and the warm brightness. That was new. It moved me. I felt goosebumps. The session was coming to an end. I asked how she felt.

"Better than when we started. When the darkness came over me, it was like I couldn't think anymore, couldn't do anything, couldn't feel anything, couldn't say anything. I was afraid something was happening that I couldn't control or explain. I didn't expect the light and warmth that came after the darkness."

"After you allowed the darkness and the coldness, you experienced something warm and bright. You began the hour with your mother's stare, where you find no place and no hold. Could it be that, in the emptiness, in the suffocating darkness in your head, and in the shock of not being able to think and feel, you are reliving some of the fear and inner darkness you felt upon not finding a place for yourself in your mother's stare?"

"I can't say yes to that, and I can't say no. Let me think about it."

The First Shared Laugh

In one of the follow-up sessions, Julia shared the following: "I no longer assume that I think the other person thinks what I am afraid of, so I have to stop that. Yesterday, I was five minutes late dropping off Mina at the kindergarten. That happens very rarely. I thought it was okay. But I deal poorly with the indirect criticism of the kindergarten teacher. She didn't address me, but Mina: 'Oh, I thought you weren't coming anymore.' I would have preferred to say, 'If Mina isn't coming, I'll call.'"

"That sounds fitting. Could you have said that?"

"No. I'm afraid that the kindergarten teacher would be mean to me, and that I'd be like a deer in the headlights."

"At least you already have a suitable phrase in store for what you *could* say."

"Mina then told me in the afternoon that she had burped extra in the presence of the childcare worker."

We both laughed heartily at this. Julia went on to say that Mina had asked, "Mom, can you burp too when you want to?" When Julia said "no," Mina showed her mother how to swallow air and then achieve the desired result. Julia's attempts to burp, albeit unsuccessful, delighted Mina. Then Julia related another experience with Mina: Recently, on a walk, Mina greeted other people in a friendly way and was pleased to be greeted back. When Julia asked why she greeted the strangers, Mina said, "I'm collecting voices."

Mina's development pleases me, and I have to think of the voice I used to address her as a baby.

A Bloody Scalp and Emerging Sadness

Julia began a session seated, "Paying attention to unpleasant things scares me. It makes me feel parched."

"Where?"

"On my scalp. Paying attention to my scalp scares me."

Again, I feel – as if dreaming – the narrative of another patient who recounted the image of her loving grandmother from the Rhineland stroking her granddaughter's head tenderly, saying, "Liebchen, your little silver hairs shine like silk." This moving moment makes me think Julia had missed out on such tenderness.

She continues, "Sometimes my scalp is so bloody that it disgusts me. I don't want anything to do with it. It's like disliking someone."

"'Someone' maybe not, but you? What about you and me together?"

I watched on the screen as she lay down on her sofa. Then she requested a familiar relaxation text from me, which I recited. After a period of silence, she said, "I feel an itchy, tingling sensation on my head. It feels tingly, spongy, mainly on the left side of the head. And on the left part from the back, below the shoulders."

I adjusted my attention to my scalp and upper back. As I did so, I observed that I involuntarily scratched the back of my head and felt a slight itch on my right shoulder. Julia then talks about rejecting helpful creams for her skin because she is afraid of becoming effeminate.

"I'd like to understand what you're saying: How do you experience being effeminate?"

"That the feeling of itching and burning and hurting is too much for me. I don't want to admit it to myself that it hurts so much." That made me so sad I felt tears coming to my eyes.

"Even just talking about it, it's already hard for me to admit to myself, to feel and think that my scalp hurts. I'd like to say 'no' every time someone asks me if my scalp hurts." The tears rising in her voice conveyed sadness.

"I think right now you're doing your skin a favor by giving space to both parts of yourself: The old part doesn't want to feel anything, and the new part feels the skin and accepts it as it is – and can become sad. I'm touched that you dare to do that."

"It scares me. In the last few days, I get sad for no reason when I'm driving. In the car, I can't distract myself from the sadness."

"I think you're growing with your sadness."

The Psychoanalytic Body Talk That Opens Up New Mental Spaces

The behavior of a 6-week-old child in response to their mother's bodily distress made a deep impression on me: a child who would not budge from her mother's side; a mother who was tormented by thoughts of her child's death. By speaking to the child while engaging the mother with my insight, I brought about a change – however explicable – that seemed to open new mental space in the child and between the mother and the child. This change initially induced separation through differentiation while simultaneously enabling a deeper connection between the mother and the child – and in the analytic relationship between the patient and myself.

Not being allowed to live and yet wanting to live against the mother's will was a conflict Julia could handle only by living "half a life": less body weight, less joy of living, and less acknowledged anger. As if to punish herself for allowing herself even that half, she lived in constant expectation of disaster in the form of her daughter's death. Guilt and the fear of punishment controlled the more mature parts of herself, which had developed the ability to symbolize. Enclosed within lay those parts that, as in a cocoon or an "encapsulated engram" (Leikert), inaccessibly harbored their unthought knowledge (Bollas, 1997 [1987]) as implicit relational knowledge. Gradually, though still only partially, this knowledge – the "secret" in her dream – became accessible and mutable. This occurred not only through free association but also through the body's sensory system and through new relational experiences in the form of mentalizing work with the bodily sensations based on a sensory-intuitive attitude – all within the matrix of presence, resonance, embodied counter-transference, transference, and resistance.

The excerpts from our psychoanalytic work presented here – experiencing one's heart rhythm and windpipe, tolerating the cold blackness in the head in which a small, warm brightness emerged for the first time, dealing with the scalp, and allowing sadness to emerge for the first time – have the role of puzzle pieces that emerged from the new encounters in the therapeutic relationship. They came together in small, slow steps to form an increasingly more solid inner representation of the body, which then became progressively more differentiated from the representation of the mother's body-self and behavior.

Toward the end of the treatment period presented above, the patient's familiarity with her bodily sensations led to their increasing transformation into emotions, primarily feelings of sadness and anger, which became more palpable. The connection between the systems of body and soul gradually grew from the work with body language, albeit not yet to the point where Julia could accept her murderous anger and connect and regulate it with her love. She and I needed to continue our path together for that to occur.

References

Anzieu, D. (1991 [1985]): *Das Haut-Ich*. Trans. by M. Korte u.M.-H. Lebourdais-Weiss. Frankfurt a. M.: Suhrkamp.

Beland, H. (2020): *Leidenschaftliches Zuhören bei namenloser Angst. Psychoanalytische Aufsätze III zu Theorie, Klinik und Gesellschaft*. Gießen: Psychosozial.

Bion, W. R. (1990 [1962]): *Lernen durch Erfahrung*. Trans. by E. Krejci. Frankfurt a. M.: Suhrkamp.

Birksted-Breen, D. (2019): Pathways of the unconscious: When the body is the receiver/ instrument. *Int J Psychoanal*, 100, 1117–1133.

Bollas, C. (1997 [1987]): *Der Schatten des Objekts. Das unbekannte Bekannte. Zur Psychoanalyse der frühen Entwicklung*. Trans. by C. Trunk. Stuttgart: Klett-Cotta.

Ferenczi, S. (1982 [1929]): Das unwillkommene Kind und sein Todestrieb. In: *Schriften zur Psychoanalyse Band II.* Frankfurt a. M.: Fischer Taschenbuch, 251–256.

Fonagy, P., Gergely, G., Jurist, E. L. & Target, M. (2004 [2002]): *Affektregulierung, Mentalisierung und die Entwicklung des Selbst.* Trans. by E. Verspohl. Stuttgart: Klett-Cotta.

Gaddini, E. (2015): Die Aktivität der kindlichen Psyche. In: Jappe, G. & Strehlow, B. (Eds.): *"Das Ich ist vor allem ein körperliches." Beiträge zur Psychoanalyse der ersten Strukturen.* Trans. by A. Jappe, exp. by L. Jappe & C. Merck-Döring. Frankfurt a. M.: Brandes & Apsel.

Gumbrecht, H. U. (2004): *Diesseits der Hermeneutik — Die Produktion von Präsenz.* Frankfurt a. M.: Suhrkamp.

Gumbrecht, H. U. (2012): *Präsenz.* Frankfurt a. M.: Suhrkamp.

Hartung, T. & Steinbrecher, M. (2018): From somatic pain to psychic pain: The body in the psychoanalytic field. *Int J Psychoanal,* 99, 159–180.

Hidas, G. & Raffai, J. (2021 [2002]): *Nabelschnur der Seele. Psychoanalytisch orientierte Förderung der vorgeburtlichen Bindung zwischen Mutter und Baby.* Trans. by N. Katschnig. Gießen: Psychosozial.

Janus, L. (2016). Die prä- und perinatale Zeit des Lebens (–9 Monate bis 0 Monate/ Geburt). In: Poscheschnik, G. & Traxl, B. (Eds.): *Handbuch Psychoanalytische Entwicklungswissenschaft.* Gießen: Psychosozial.

Kobylinska-Dehe, E. (2019): Vom Leib zum phantasmatischen Körper – Bewegung, Berührung, Phantasie. *Psyche – Z Psychoanal,* 73, 523–545. 10.21706-Psyche-73-7

Küchenhoff, J. (2012): *Körper und Sprache. Theoretische und klinische Beiträge zu einem intersubjektiven Verständnis des Körpererlebens.* Gießen: Psychosozial.

Leikert, S. (2019): *Das sinnliche Selbst. Das Körpergedächtnis in der psychoanalytischen Behandlungstechnik.* Frankfurt a. M.: Brandes & Apsel.

Lemma, A. (2018 [2015]): *Der Körper spricht immer. Körperlichkeit in psychoanalytischen Therapien und jenseits der Couch.* Trans. by L. Apsel. Frankfurt a. M.: Brandes & Apsel.

Lempa, G. (2021): Neuere Entwicklungen in der psychoanalytischen Psychosentherapie. *Psyche – Z Psychoanal,* 75, 4–39.

Leuzinger-Bohleber, M. (2009): *Frühe Kindheit als Schicksal? Trauma, Embodiment, Soziale Desintegration. Psychoanalytische Perspektiven.* Stuttgart: Kohlhammer.

Leuzinger-Bohleber, M., Emde, R. N. & Pfeifer, R. (Eds.) (2013): *Embodiment. Ein innovatives Konzept für Entwicklungsforschung und Psychoanalyse.* Göttingen: Vandenhoeck & Ruprecht.

Lombardi, R. (2019): Mysteries, abysses, and impasses in body-mind dissociation. *Int J Psychoanal,* 100, 1371–1389.

Lombardi, R. (2021 [2019]): Die Dissoziation von Körper und Psyche – Rätsel, Abgründe und Sackgassen. In: Münch, K. (Ed.): *Internationale Psychoanalyse,* 16, 257–283. Gießen: Psychosozial.

Ogden, T. O. (1995 [1989]): *Frühe Formen des Erlebens.* Trans. by H. Friessner & E.-M. Wolfram. Wien/New York: Springer.

Plassmann, R. (2019): *Psychotherapie der Emotionen. Die Bedeutung von Emotionen für die Entstehung und Behandlung von Krankheiten.* Gießen: Psychosozial.

Raffai, J. (2008): Mündliche Mitteilung.

Rank, O. (1924): *Das Trauma der Geburt und seine Bedeutung für die Psychoanalyse.* Neuausgabe (1988) Frankfurt a. M.: Fischer.

Scharff, J. M. (2010): *Die leibliche Dimension in der Psychoanalyse.* Frankfurt a. M.: Brandes & Apsel.

Schmidt, M. G. (2014): Der Einfluss der Präsenztheorie auf die psychoanalytische Behandlungstechnik. *Psyche – Z Psychoanal*, 68, 951–970.

Schore, A. N. (2009): *Affektregulation und die Reorganisation des Selbst*. Trans. by E. Rass. Stuttgart: Klett-Cotta.

Schultz-Venrath, U. (2021): *Mentalisieren des Körpers*. Stuttgart: Klett-Cotta.

Schultz-Venrath, U. & Felsberger, H. (2016): *Mentalisieren in Gruppen*. Stuttgart: Klett-Cotta.

Stern, D. N. (2014 [2004]): *Der Gegenwartsmoment. Veränderungsprozesse in Psychoanalyse, Psychotherapie und Alltag*. Trans. by E. Vorspohl. Frankfurt a. M.: Brandes & Apsel. 5th ed. 2018.

Stern, D. N. et al. (The Boston Change Process Study Group) (2012 [2010]): *Veränderungsprozesse. Ein integratives Paradigma*. Übers.: E. Vorspohl. Frankfurt a. M.: Brandes & Apsel. 2nd ed. 2021.

Storck, T. (2016): *Psychoanalyse und Psychosomatik. Die leiblichen Grundlagen der Psychosomatik*. Stuttgart: Kohlhammer.

Terry, K. (2008–2012): Babytherapy courses. Mündliche Mitteilungen im Weiterbildungskurs.

Volz-Boers, U. (1999): "Ich bin wieder ein Mensch." Transformation des frühen psychischen Traumas durch Neubildung von Repräsentanzen. *Psyche – Z Psychoanal*, 53, 1138–1159.

Volz-Boers, U. (2016): Resonanz im Körper des Analytikers. Das Konzept der sensorischintuitiven Haltung. In: Walz-Pawlita, S., Unruh, B. & Janta, B. (Eds.): *Körper-Sprachen*. Gießen: Psychosozial, 141–152.

Warsitz, P. (2014). Indirekte Symbolisierung in poetischer Sprache. *Psyche – Z Psychoanal*, 68, S. 840–865.

Wolf, K., Lan, F. & Wallner, F. (Eds.) (2018): *Präsenztherapie. Neue psychotherapeutische Implikationen im Wandel des abendländischen und des fernöstlichen Denkens*. Stuttgart: Thieme.

Chapter 8

Mind the Gap
Mentalizing the Body

Ulrich Schultz-Venrath

For some time now, psychoanalysts and psychodynamic psychotherapists as well as molecular biologists,[1] neuroscientists, and attachment researchers have shown an increased interest in affect and emotion. This is expressed in refreshing but often disparate concepts of how to better understand the role and importance of the body in the psychotherapy of a wide variety of disorders – not just somatoform stress disorders. Examples are Sebastian Leikert (2019), Alessandra Lemma (2014), Riccardo Lombardi (2008, 2017), Reinhard Plassmann (1993, 2019), Jörg Scharff (2010), Ulla Volz-Boers (2004, 2007, 2009), and others, who have increasingly placed the various facets of bodily phenomena or even the body itself at the center of their treatment techniques.[2] In the process, they overlooked or failed to cite many earlier pioneers, such as Didier Anzieu (2016 [1991]), Eugenio Gaddini (1998 [1981]), Gisela Pankow (1974), or Joyce McDougall (1991), and quite a few others because the body plays a rather disruptive role in psychoanalysis. All of these researchers, however, are united by the recognition that psychic activity follows bodily activity (and not vice versa), and that this basic somatopsychic organization makes the cohesion of the subject possible in the first place, like some protective skin that holds the self and object parts together while simultaneously keeping them separate from the outside world. Eugenio Gaddini was firmly convinced that "physiological learning necessarily precedes psychological learning. As long as the fetal state continues, this sequence can be seen as the original expression of the body-psyche-function continuum [...] that precedes birth" (Gaddini, 1998 [1981], p. 25). In our view, the body-psyche-function continuum dominates postnatally, at least until the ninth month of life. It plays a significant role throughout life as a "body-mode" when we resort to in the prementalistic mode regarding affect regulation. Only with the onset of the psychological function of skin, the extremities, or the body as boundaries do representations of the body-self, the body-fantasies, or fantasies in the body occur and can be accessed through language. Like speech development, however, the path to this juncture is long and rocky in the sense of body development and developmental psychology.

DOI: 10.4324/9781003370130-8

Despite the multitude of body psychotherapies – Wikipedia lists 28 different representatives under this keyword – the mentalizing model is presently proving to be particularly productive scientifically: Despite differing basic scientific assumptions, it can integrate the most diverse disciplines regarding essential somatopsychic functions, such as developmental biology and neurobiology, affect and autism research as well as attachment research, including various body-friendly psychoanalytic concepts. Just in passing, meta-analytically, mentalizing-based individual and group psychotherapy (MBT/ MBT-G) has emerged as the most effective long-term psychotherapy method to treat borderline personality disorder (Storebo et al., 2020) – and this patient group suffers from not a few body complaints.

The potpourri of previous analytic body psychotherapy literature has a flaw regarding scientific theory: Out of ignorance of historical antecedents and the broad literature, scientific complexity regarding representational, affective, and memory theory is avoided in favor of more salient solutions. Yet simplification does not necessarily make them more correct. Sometimes the impression arises that the body conception propagated in each case is due more to the life history of the respective author, for instance, as a physician or psychologist, including the specialist orientation (gynecology, psychiatry, neurology, pediatrics) or analytic origin (Winnicott, Lacan, Klein, Bion, etc.), which is, however, rarely revealed (Kuchuck, 2013). As a representative of the mentalizing model, I therefore freely confess – in addition to my analytic training in the German DPV – my loyalty to my neurophysiological and neurological teacher, Dieter Janz, a disciple of Viktor von Weizsäcker and an epileptologist who felt connected to psychosomatic neurology (Strzelczyk & Schmitt, 2020), long before I met Peter Fonagy in 1996 during the first Research Summer School Training at the University College London (UCL). My group-analytic training, which introduced me to S. H. Foulkes and his neurological teacher, Kurt Goldstein, both Jewish émigrés, deepened my understanding of the body in terms of its sociocultural embeddedness, which his student Patrick DeMaré expressed in the sentence: "I think with my feelings and feel my thoughts."[3]

Less well known is that, even in the early days of psychoanalysis, there was a great interest in the body, not the least because of the mass occurrence of war neuroses in the First World War. Fierce controversies among psychoanalysts, psychotherapists, and psychiatrists accompanied the question of the theory and treatment of the body because the theory of the etiopathogenesis of sexual conflicts in war-neurotic conversion disorders could no longer be sustained (Alexander, 1948; Deutsch, 1926; Ferenczi, 1919; Schröter, 2018; Schultz-Venrath, 1995 [1992]; Simmel, 1918). Simmel and Ferenczi understood traumatic neuroses as the severe regression into a phylogenetic and ontogenetic "proto-psyche" in which "states of excitement [...] are simply managed by motor discharge" (Ferenczi, 1919 [1984], p. 184). Beginning in 1916, the mass occurrence of war neuroses and the simultaneous failure of psychiatric galvanic electro-treatment methods catapulted psychoanalysts such as Karl Abraham, Sandor Ferenczi, and Ernst Simmel to the forefront in war-neurosis hospitals, a health policy success of short duration for psychoanalysis. Even then, the reflections of individual psychoanalysts regarding the body and its disorders went beyond the Freudian concept of conversion to address the unsatisfactory psychophysical parallelism and the dichotomization of the body-soul problem from a scientific and epistemological standpoint. But almost all authors adhered to the drive theory and the role of the "psyche," thus maintaining the schism. Anna Margaretha Stegmann (1926, pp. 197 f.), for example, expressed that it was "logical for psychoanalysis to regard the soul (spirit) as primary [...]", which is why "the soul [...] is the meaning of [i.e., the reason for] the body" and "the body is [...] the expression of the soul." Ernst Simmel, on the other hand, followed Karl Abraham and attempted to bridge the gap from the human body to psychoanalysis by proposing an "intestinal libido" that emerges postnatally, thereby assigning to the digestive tract – as the earliest stage of libido development – the "stimulus reception, stimulus distribution, and stimulus discharge." In this scenario, the digestive tract simultaneously connects and separates the psyche and the soma (Schultz-Venrath & Hermanns, 2019; Simmel, 1924). That most psychoanalysts more or less lost sight of the body as the very foundation of all psychic development likely goes back to their enthusiasm for the psychic. But even Paul Schilder (1978 [1935], p. 201) knew that we act "in every action [...] not only as persons but also with our bodies."

However, the juxtaposition of the various psychodynamic theories of the body and its phenomena effectively continues the tradition of scientific subjectivism or individualism, something Viktor von Weizsäcker (1954, p. 125) had already criticized about Freud and his view of psychoanalysis. It ultimately goes back to a hitherto incompatible understanding of science – hermeneutic versus empirical. Thus, to this day, the psychodynamic literature contains numerous, sometimes rather adventurous, fantasies or attributions to bodily phenomena, such as the recent attribution of trichotillomania and trichotillophagia to cannibalistic impulses (Schiller, 2021). Such ideas point more toward the therapist's rather than the patient's deep-set fantasies. In developmental psychology, it is now undisputed that, in addition to secure attachment, affect regulation plays a central role in the development of self and object representations. Like all other living beings, the infant enters the world with a set of innate needs. The stages of psychic development formulated by Freud – "oral," "anal," and "genital" – already pointed to the physical needs that dominate during early childhood. However, the somatic origin of these terms, which marked the so-called libido stages, has been largely lost through their predominantly metapsychological application, although Freud, in his account of the succession of erogenous zones, also designed a model for structuring affective bodily experience. Likewise, it is largely forgotten today that the drive concept "as a concept of the boundary between the psychic and the somatic" (Freud, 1915c, p. 214) at its core implied the somatization of the psychic in psychoanalysis. Basic emotions trigger instinctive behaviors that can be traced back to innate action plans, which are executed to meet the respective needs (such as crying, seeking, fleeing, attacking). However, to date, no general agreement has been reached on the nature and number of innate needs.

In psychotherapies, the patient's body, which may be unloved, hated, or associated with pain, is present in the (bodily) countertransference more often than some therapists would like to admit. This occurs because of how we therapists tend to listen to the body and its stories – and here I largely follow Alessandra Lemma (2014): We are both theoretically and practically influenced by our subjectivity (encompassing bodily and psychological elements), i.e., our experiences with our own body, its affects, and emotions.

The Body in the Mentalizing-Based Initial Interview

The initial conversation is by no means just a conversation. It is "only" the tip of an iceberg that contains a multitude of actions embedded into therapeutic efficacy or inefficacy (Schmidt, 2019). The initial interview differs depending on the level of training (biopsychosocial, psychiatric, or psychoanalytic), location (clinic, day clinic, practice), the therapist's conscious and unconscious interest (holistic, descriptive, or in terms of an operationalized psychodynamic diagnosis – OPD). After the greeting, the first mentalizing-based question – "How do you feel?" – immediately brings the body and its state of being into focus, to which some patients respond with the counterquestion, "Do you mean now or before?" It is worthwhile telling patients that they can decide what they want to talk about and what is important to them. It is all about joint or shared attention, whereby the therapist tries to see the patient's world through the patient's eyes and not just as a gestalt via "scenic understanding" and listening (Buchholz, 2020). At the same time, the "interviewer" must consider epistemic mistrust when ensuring an offer of a "secure relationship," providing it only piecemeal to patients with an insecure or even disorganized attachment style stemming from early neglect or traumatization. In this respect, the first step is clarifying together how intercorporeal trust can be established in the first place. Most patients with bodily symptoms have never had a secure bond, or it may feel threatening to them. Not infrequently, they react with withdrawal and terminate the analysis. Video analyses of initial interviews, even those of trained and experienced therapists, impressively demonstrate that the first meeting can be much more challenging to implement than expected. Out of uncertainty, analysts may pose closed questions instead of open ones, causing mentalizing to come to a standstill.

In contrast to the initial analytic interview, the MBT therapist does not suggest to the patient that they can talk about anything on their mind during the next 50 minutes. In contrast, the silent analyst continues to write everything down, their gaze directed toward the paper in front of them. Also, the sitting posture – leaning forward rather than leaning back – seems to affect the ability to mentalize. Often the first questions are different – or even several questions are asked at the same time, which signal a counter-transference resistance and do not help engender an authentic relationship with the patient.

The initial psychosomatic and psychoanalytic interviews use the first-person perspective to concentrate on self-experience rather than feelings and affects reflected in bodily experiences. Although, to be clear, there is no such thing as a non-body-self (Henningsen, 2021) – as if the body (Körper/Leib) has not yet found its rightful place, linguistically or methodologically. This is also reflected in the perceptions of therapists who, from a second-person perspective, tend to pinpoint the conflict level or self-structure. We find this, among other things, in the system of Operationalized Psychodynamic Diagnostic (OPD2), whether in terms of interpersonal behavior regarding the other person and oneself, or in terms of how it refers to the patient's experience of illness. The latter is only of interest inasmuch as it is a somatic, factor-oriented concept of illness (Arbeitskreis-OPD, 2014).

The initial interview or case history begins with the voice on the answering machine, before the first direct contact at the practice door. Unfortunately, there is no systematic research available on the role of the therapist's voice on their answering machines and on whether the respective patient even wants to get in touch with a therapist who speaks in this way or that – and even less is available on the fantasies the therapist's voice may trigger. In the prepandemic era, in addition to what the visual and olfactory senses could gather, the handshake still played a special role in the initial encounter, which the therapist could experience as either soft, rubbery, limp, and powerless, or sometimes as too brisk, forced, even painfully aggressive. Hands can be cold or hot, dry or moist, hard or soft, all of which are physical, preverbal signals, like when two hands fail to meet. No less effective, but little addressed, are tattoos that suddenly appear on the neck, arm, and leg, fulfilling the patient's bodily need for solidity, a sense of stability, and a means of indelible expression (Karacaoğlan, 2012). Corporeality, intercorporeity, and embodiment all refer to bodily exchanges in the "in-between," which is more or less congruent with what Stern calls the "implicit relationship" (Schmidt, 2020).

When infants are exposed relatively early on, in part prenatally, to the internal patterns of physiological and visceral stimulations, postnatally they learn to discriminate in their own bodies by scanning the facial expression and voice of the primary caregiver and how the latter reacts to the expression of their inner processes. It is fair to assume that this applies quite similarly to the patient–therapist relationship: The categorization of faces occurs within 100 milliseconds, and the specific recognition of individual identity, i.e., of the body, takes no more than 170 milliseconds (Adolphs, 2003). Somewhat slower, but no less impressive, this phenomenon was empirically verified in experienced clinicians who were shown videotaped initial conversations in small "portions" of 1 minute each. After only 3 minutes, clinicians could formulate diagnoses that did not change significantly after receiving further information from a 1-hour interview (Schwartz & Wiggins, 1987). Wegner and Henseler (1991) made similar observations regarding the description of the very first scene in an initial interview up until the patient's first sentence. They studied a group of analytically trained colleagues who were asked to formulate a psychodynamic diagnosis – which turned out to be accurate – based on the recorded scene, oriented toward body movements and expressions. We ourselves had similar experiences with medical students in psychosomatic medicine classes using videotaped initial interviews: The students' task was to analyze the first 60 seconds of the videotaped anamnesis, first without sound, later then with sound, between a student and a patient regarding certain parameters (affects and gestures in the patient as well as in the student and affects and emotions in the student observers of the video). Under a moderation that focused the discussion on the parameters mentioned above, the medical students succeeded quite aptly in making the correct diagnosis solely based on a meticulous video analysis of the first minute without sound, albeit including the emotional reactions of the students observing the video. Finally, when the first minute of the video was played with sound, the patient's spoken words more often contradicted the observation of affective facial expressions and gestures, so the students got an impression of observing an unconscious defense of an already diagnosed unconscious expression or even conflict based on the patient's facial expression, gestures, and movement (Schultz-Venrath, 2015 [2013]).

These examples indicate that, even in interactions with a narrow temporal scope, an implicit, preconscious, mimetically contingent relational knowledge develops, presumably based on a preconceptual representation. "Preconceptual means: it is visible and perceptible on the video recording to third parties but not to the participant" (Buchholz, 2003, p. 37). Buchholz prefers the term "preconceptual" because "representation" already presupposes a separation between two people, whereas here we are dealing with a mimetic connection that *precedes* the separation and makes the interaction possible in the first place. Perhaps the concept of a functional – nonstatic – protomental representation would also be helpful in this regard. Merleau-Ponty (1974 [1965]) attempted to grasp this phenomenon using the concept of "intercorporeity," whereas the British psychologist Colwyn Trevarthen (1979; Trevarthen & Aitken, 2001) suggested "primary intersubjectivity," which for the embryo already begins in the womb between mother and embryo as a sort of "musical" communication. Sandler and Sandler (1984) preferred the alternative "present unconscious."

Despite these observations, these processes are highly individual and depend on numerous factors, such as voice pitch or the particular sitting position: A therapist who leans forward displays embodied interest and an attitude of curiosity for the narrative of the counterpart. This is significant because patients with certain mental and psychosomatic disorders, such as borderline (BPD) or antisocial personality disorder, are characterized by, among other things, their difficulty in correctly interpreting facial expressions. While patients with autism spectrum disorder tend to fixate their counterparts' eyes less, BPD patients seem to be highly sensitive and react to emotional facial expressions "without warning" – indeed, much faster than healthy individuals (Lynch et al., 2006). This can lead to insinuations and misconceptions, such as when a supervisor unexpectedly fails to say "hello" and a BPD patient interprets this to mean that the supervisor does not like them, though it was likely just an inattention on the part of the supervisor. Delinquent adolescents are also poor at interpreting emotional facial expressions, for example, misinterpreting disgust in the other person as anger (Sato et al., 2009). These misinterpretations are not limited to visual effects but may also affect the interoception controlled by the insula, which helps the body maintain the physiological framework needed for its functions.

The importance of this region, which lies below the temporal lobe, was discovered by the Canadian neurosurgeons Penfield and Faulk (1955) when, during a partial temporal lobectomy under partial anesthesia in patients with pharmacoresistant temporal lobe epilepsy, they induced strange sensations in the abdomen or stomach, dizziness, or nausea. Neurobiologically, the insula is saddled with multiple tasks, the most significant (and vulnerable) of which seems to be the processing of signals from inside the body. Thus, severe childhood maltreatment leads to sensory dysregulation in the right somato-sensory cortex, posterior insular region, and hippocampus, which in experiments manifests in preferences for greater interpersonal distance and negative responses to social touch (Maier et al., 2020). In addition, reduced oxytocin receptors are found in the mononuclear cells of persons who experienced maltreatment during childhood (Krause et al., 2018). This may explain, at least in part, why individuals with severe childhood maltreatment often have difficulty both forming and maintaining closer social bonds later in life. It also helps us to better understand the sudden breakdown of their fragile self-structure under psychosocial stress.

Regarding visual perception, facial expressions are again of utmost relevance, because the intensity of synchronization between mother and child during first 10 years of life determines the extent of the child's later capacity for empathy (Levy & Feldman, 2019). Empathy is by no means an automatic process but rather grows out of an intentional stance, even though mirror neurons governing imitative skills might suggest this. Nor is it a reflex: It is a developmental *achievement* (Solms, 2021, p. 326). Thus, it is not surprising that various illnesses display disturbances in the synchronization of body movements with an interaction partner, each in their own specific way regarding empathic ability. The most serious occur apparently in hospitalized patients with schizophrenic psychoses (Krause, 1992). However, body synchronization phenomena are notably absent when the patient lies on the couch.

Noncontingencies or missing synchronizations are also significant for the development of mentalizing at the protomental, self-structural level. From about the third month of life, infants seem to know that anything not perfectly contingent on their own actions does not belong to them. So, they begin to look for imperfect contingencies and discover them in the noncontingent mimicry (and physical) response of the primary attachment figure (usually the mother) to their affective expressions. Yet, it is unclear to what extent this can be incorporated into therapeutic processes. Interestingly, therapists who allow the patient to "control" their own facial expressions, i.e., who allow themselves to be affectively "infected" and who only copy the patient's facial expressions, achieve worse treatment results than those who are more differentiated in their affect expressions and sometimes react antithetically toward the patient (Krause, 1992). The interactions of such therapists reflect noncontingent mirroring by displaying a certain differential, i.e., the therapist does not show sadness when the patient is sad but exhibits appropriate mimicry expressing "concern" or even hidden aspects of the feeling. Affects are intentional and express a "desire for altered object relations" or a "continuation of object relations" (Krause, 1992, p. 599). All of this plays a role even before and during the initial interview, which is occasionally subsumed somewhat too sweepingly and undifferentiated under the term "embodiment."

In the subsequent psychotherapy as well, therapists should listen to more than just the spoken word, specifically to the emotional tone (which is based on expressions suitable to communicate affects while not always representing an affect), to rhythm, prosody, and mimic expression. Of course, it is difficult to perceive one's own physical and psychological processes and those of the patient at the same time. The trick lies in including as many senses as possible – the visual, the tactile, and the olfactory – and not just what the patient *says*. This entails entering into an authentic relationship with the patient, reserving one's interpretations but offering affect-focused, curious, and sometimes surprising questions based on one's perceptions. The therapist's ability to initially put a positive twist on a negative affect seems to be particularly effective in this regard (Isen et al., 1987). In addition to mastering theory, self-awareness, and supervision, the therapist must practice this approach again and again via video recordings or role plays, in the sense of experiential learning as the fourth pillar of training, to determine which type of intervention or interaction better fits the patient in which situation (Ehrenthal, 2019; Scharff, 2021). If we define psychotherapy as the attempt to develop new perspectives by forming new representations, the therapist requires a special presence to make this happen. "Corporeality, intercorporeity, and embodiment emphasize the bodily relatedness of actions; they make intelligible the extremely bodily organized forms of memory in which sensomotor elements of action play a central role. Here one can no longer deny the nonrepressed, implicit-unconscious level." (Schmidt, 2020)

In this respect, the mentalizing model of Fonagy and his research group (Fonagy et al., 2002 [2004]) represents a (radical) extension of the basic psychoanalytic concept. It integrates empirical findings on attachment and affect research as well as trauma and the neurosciences. Although the body does not appear in the concept of mentalizing itself, mentalizing is by no means "only" a mental process; it is a concept that reflects the borderline between soma and psyche: Mentalizing as a processual module of the regulation of early bodily and affective experiences cannot be thought of without considering the body. *Mentalizing cannot take place without the body!* Mentalizing begins with the body and is experienced through the body. The mentalizing model goes hand in hand with a revival of the integration of body and psyche, of body and mind. What is especially interesting, however, are the culturally determined differences regarding the relative importance of the body, as they have developed historically in France, England, and Germany, which are also reflected in subtly different theoretical concepts of mentalizing.

Knowing the four prementalizing modes of affect regulation (Table 8.1) and the four dimensions of mentalizing is very helpful: implicit versus explicit, cognitive versus affective, internally oriented versus externally oriented, and self versus other. Each of them requires a different technique (Schultz-Venrath, 2021) to promote mentalizing in both the patient and the therapist. A psychotherapist can fall into a prementalistic mode from which they, like the patient, can best emerge through countermovements ("contrary moves") (Schultz-Venrath, 2021, p. 192). Of all the prementalistic modes, the body-mode and the teleological mode are most closely associated with implicit memory (Figure 8.1). Clinically, the body-mode is the most widespread, appearing in the form of thumb-sucking, skin-picking, self-injury of all kinds,

Table 8.1 Definition of prementalistic modes (Schultz-Venrath, 2021)

Mode	Description
Body	Pre- and postnatal the baby cannot experience body and psyche separately until around the ninth month. He/she is *primarily concerned with his/her body and skin* sensations. The body-mode is self-oriented.
Teleological	Mental states such as needs and emotions are expressed in action. The environment must "function" in order to alleviate one's own inner states of tension. Understanding of others in terms of physical behaviors. *Only actions* and their available consequences count – not words. The teleological mode is object-oriented.
Equivalent	*Outer world = inner world.* Mental states are experienced as real, as happens in dreams, flashbacks, and paranoid delusions.
Pretend	Mental states are disconnected from reality, retain a *sense of unreality* because they are not connected and anchored to reality

Memory, modes of affect -regulation & language

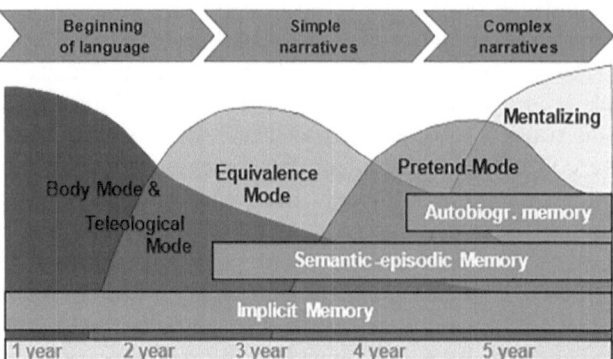

Figure 8.1 Prementalistic modes relative to language development and memory.

dermatillomania, tattoos, hyperembodiment in eating disorders, nail-biting (onychophagia), nailbed-biting (perionychophagia), body-focused repetitive behavior disorders, psychogenic seizures, vaginismus, priapism, hypersexuality, bodybuilding, and most recently the increasing use of self-tracking (using a smartwatch to measure daily steps taken, heart rate, and much more). But dentists are also familiar with the phenomenon of occlusal dysesthesia, when patients complain of persistent discomfort and pain because of awkwardly perceived tooth contact, often after a difficult dental procedure. Like the most common body-mode symptoms, they can be viewed as both an attempt at self-reassurance and an unconscious attack on the self-concept when self and object representations are unstable. Patients in body-mode perceive "mental states" only as physiological–bodily sensations and express them automatically because of innate tendencies.

Vignette of a Mentalizing-Based Initial Interview

A 68-year-old, hearing-impaired, rather lonely female patient reports a harsh rejection after attempting to contact a female friend (a writer) with whom she had had a 30-year friendship. Following the death of her husband (25 years her elder) 3 years ago, the friend had broken off contact, disappointed that the patient had not cared enough for her when her husband was dying. At about the same time, she – the patient – had heard a "motor noise, starting over and over again" in her apartment. She had called the building management and contacted the more than 80 other residents in the building to find out the source of the noise, until it turned out that it was tinnitus. When I asked her exactly where she was hearing the tinnitus, she replied, "It vibrates through my whole body" (a differential to tinnitus aureum, by the way!). Surprisingly, however, this sensation only occurs indoors. Asked whether this noise has any connection to her feeling alive, she laughed with a snort and said, well, she had felt more alive again after contacting all the fellow residents of the building. Alone the diagnosis of tinnitus, she said, made the symptomatology much weaker.

Can Mentalizing Take Place on the Couch?

The couch (formerly: the divan, the sofa, or the chaise longue) has become an established cultural symbol in the media and cartoons from psychodynamic procedures. The first duty of candidates training to be analysts in continuing education institutions is still reaching a high level of self-experience. This means that, by nature, they have insufficient own experience not only with bodily phenomena but also with the meaning and effect of low-frequency therapies. Patients with bodily complaints and/or somatoform stress disorders usually do not initially present to a psychoanalyst, a psychotherapist, a psychosomatic therapist, or a psychiatrist. Instead, they usually first visit their primary-care physician, a neurologist, or the emergency room. Although their physicians may occasionally intuitively ponder the possibility of functional complaints in certain constellations ("I had the feeling right away that something wasn't adding up"), the "road to the couch" is long: First, an extensive and expensive diagnostic regimen to exclude all other possibilities must be worked through despite any initial intuition. Publications relating a successful psychoanalytic or psychosomatic couch treatment of patients with somatization disorders, such as that of Marie Cardinal (1979), are the exceptions that confirm the rule.

The microanalytic findings of attachment research (Beebe et al., 2019), the new rationale of affect research (Krause, 1992; Panksepp, 2009; Panksepp & Biven, 2012), and the growth of neuropsychoanalytic findings regarding the emergence of consciousness (Solms, 2021) – which turns the Freudian concept of the cortical seat of the ego on its head – are not very compatible with previous psychoanalytic theories or classical practice. Nor are they sufficiently compatible with the sweeping notion of "embodiment" that made its triumph in cognitive psychology with the book *The Embodied Mind* (Varela et al., 2016 [1991]). Not only the mirror neurons, which play a major role in unconscious imitative behaviors, but also the brainstem have the greatest impact on primary affects. Jaak Panksepp empirically proved there are seven basal emotions (SEEKING, PLAY [JOY], CARE [LOVE], LUST [SEXUAL], FEAR/PANIC [separation distress], and RAGE; Panksepp & Biven, 2012). More than anyone before him, he espoused an "affect-centered" view of mental processes and understood affects as evolutionarily conserved core physical routines underlying mental processes. His belief that basal emotions were something much more fundamental than an interesting "coloring" of the neural bases of consciousness stood – and still stands – in stark contrast to the cognition-based and predominantly sensory view of consciousness (Watt, 2017). Panksepp and Biven (2012) provided empirical evidence that affects are largely located in the brainstem and subcortical circuits and are responsible for cognitive development through neocortical circuits, something Mark Solms (2021) further differentiated.

Clinical case presentations make it apparent that bodily intersubjectivity is rarely appreciated, if at all. One reason may lie in the challenging complexity of integrating evidence from diverse sciences. Another aspect of the limited, or even missing, perception of bodily phenomena could stem from the rigid adherence of analysts to the analytic couch setting, which is still taken for granted to ensure the "corporate identity" of psychoanalysis as well as analytic training institutes – despite the decreasing number of patients being treated analytically (currently 5%). Krause's (1992, p. 610) criticism that, "from an ethological point of view, the analytical setting, especially classical analysis, […] induces shame and reduces autonomy" got a surprisingly meager reaction. It is now a truism that all negative affects inhibit mentalizing. Few psychoanalysts have critically addressed the significance of intersubjective bodily processes on the couch. Similarly, it is a desideratum that we need more scientific research on the effectiveness of teaching analysis on the couch: There are no investigations into whether regression is even useful or necessary for "successful" treatment. Regarding our patients, Leikert (2021, p. 671) rightly writes:

> In psychoanalytic work, we invite our analysands to follow up on thoughts and ideas occurring to them while reclining on the couch, where they can devote themselves to this task in a state of complete relaxation. But this is precisely what they do not do. They stay all tensed up and lie there in contorted postures as if the couch were a minefield. Intuitively, we grasp the fact that this dysregulation contains a message associ- ated with disasters in the relationship with the primary object. But how can we read this message? What language is it couched in? What roles do body-self and body-memory play in our analyses?

How did this scientistic misunderstanding come about? More than 100 years ago, Freud used the couch to create the best possible treatment method, albeit embedded in a very different sociocultural history. The couch model originated in the setting of suggestion and hypnosis, which reflected the asymmetry between analyst and patient prescribed there. Yet little attention has been paid to the risk inherent to the couch setting, where the analyst sits *behind* the patient, largely without contact with the patient's body, indeed usually in contact only by listening, sometimes by smell. Because of the patient's prone position and the analyst's sitting position, the two bodies are arranged asymmetrically, with different lines of sight: The analyst needs merely to turn their gaze slightly to observe the reclining patient, whereas the patient must resort to contortions to see the analyst. (This disregards the fact that, in some schools, the analyst may occasionally sit with their armchair visible to the patient or next to the couch. However, that contradicts Freud's original idea.) The couch anchored an emblematic asymmetry of observing and knowing. The body, with all its senses (except hearing) was largely excluded and no longer a relevant component in the psychoanalytic setting. Freud famously cited two reasons to justify his "technical" innovation: First, he preferred to sit behind his patient because he did not want to be stared at for hours. In other words, the asymmetrical position of doctor and patient serves to *avoid* visual communication, although today we can assume with some certainty that the sense of sight is the most significant of all the senses for the development of representations: "While listening, I leave myself to the course of my unconscious thoughts and do not want my facial expressions to give patients material for interpretations or influence them in their communications [...]." Second, the patient's lying on the couch serves to "isolate the transference" and "prevent the imperceptible intermingling of the transference with the patient's ideas." He thought suppressing motor actions increases the capacity for reflection (Freud, 1913c, p. 467). Consequently, the patient should only "remember" and not "interact." Thus, the spatially intervening body is conceived "primarily as imagined and in its peculiar function as a generator of fantasies" (Storck, 2021, p. 13).

This rather cognitively oriented stance, which gives preference to thinking and remembering over other sensory perceptions, has since been thoroughly overhauled by research into mirror neurons: Only the *observation* of another person (e.g., the therapist) triggers the mirror neurons to lift a stored action program to the inner imagination. This is true not only for motor action sequences but also for the sequences of feeling and sensation. Moreover, the mirror neuron system plays a fundamental role in imitation and mimicry (Bauer, 2005; Di Cesare et al., 2016; Rizzolatti et al., 1999; Rizzolatti & Sinigaglia, 2016). In this respect, not only are completely different "transference processes" formed by the supine setting, but, regarding the inter-subjective exchange at the mirror neuron level, it also results in different representational developments than sitting opposite one another – all of which are not reflected in the relevant literature. The mentalizing model, therefore, prefers to speak of "mentalizing the relationship."

Modern affect and emotion research, especially in the observation of infants, has produced many significant findings that the couch setting is indeed questionable as a therapeutic approach for the large group of patients with persistent physical complaints, for example, somatoform stress disorders or functional body complaints. There is no empirical basis to determine for whom the couch might be suitable and when free association is advantageous (Lingiardi & Dei Bei, 2011; Schachter & Kächele, 2010). Ludwig-Körner (2015) offered a similar critique regarding infant observation, where abstinence on the part of the observer of the mother–baby dyad may well prove to be traumatic for the infant if the observer does not behave resonantly toward the mother–baby dyad.

The couch setting has caused the mental expressions of a patient to be taken more seriously than the (physical) reactions of both participants, if one disregards the relatively small number of psychoanalysts who have tried – however differently – to solve this problem (Pflichthofer, 2008; Plassmann, 1993; Scharff, 2010; Volz-Boers, 2001). Even if the couch can indeed promote a specific therapeutic means of identity formation, today it is certainly questionable whether it offers a *better* path to understanding implicit-unconscious, affective-emotional bodily processes than working on unconscious fantasies. Perhaps some psychoanalysts need the couch as a place to "hide behind" (Lemma, 2018, p. 52), something they are extremely reluctant to admit. Maybe this is why large parts of the analytic "community" take the couch setting as a given, as "normal," and only recently have devoted more conceptual attention to the body in psychoanalysis.

Classically working psychoanalysts object, saying that, while lying on the couch, the patient may use their remaining senses to perceive the analyst, and that the absence of visual support may in fact favor the awareness of bodily experiences. However, this presupposes that the patient has a sufficient ability to apply the "transference object" (Quinodoz, 2003, 2011). Maybe the other senses of hearing and smelling would even be reinforced adjunctively; in the meantime, however, seeing and sense of sight have taken clear predominance over the other senses regarding the formation of representations – not the least because of cultural developments.

The container function of words may tempt some psychodynamically oriented therapists to prefer patients lie on the couch (Lemma, 2014, p. 19). Yet patients whose psychological and psychosomatic symptomatology resulted from the absence of self and object, or insufficiently stable representations thereof, need the therapist's face, facial expressions, and gaze. They object to the asymmetry by saying, "I need a counterpart – it won't work without." If we assume that somatoform disorders result either from a lack of integration of sensory and bodily experiences, in which the body imposed itself concretely, or from the body being completely split off for whatever reasons, the mutual, visible, and perceptible (!) exchange with the affective bodily reactions of the therapist as a model helps to better assign one's own perceptions. The prospect of lying on the couch often triggers in patients with somatoform disorders the fear of being overwhelmed by their diffuse affects and being unable to regulate them. However, the visible (!) exchange of the patient with the affective reactions of the therapist favors the development of new mental representations, because therapists, among other things, also represent a model of affect regulation. Numerous observations and empirical findings now recognize the therapist's authentic bodily affective responses as significant for the representational formation of affect and emotion in patients with a wide range of disorders (Krause, 2016).

The Body-Mode During MBT Supervision

A psychoanalyst reports on a 21-year-old patient, a "girl" really, with atypical anorexia and obsessive–compulsive disorder, whom she had initially treated as an inpatient for 2 years and who now comes regularly to her practice. Despite her best efforts, the analyst says, the patient "cannot find a way to speak," which means the therapist does most of the talking – and feels increasingly uncomfortable about it. Therefore, she suggests a body therapy ("somatic experience"), with which she had had a good experience. But the patient rejects it after a short time, first because the costs were too high, but also because she absolutely wants to stay with the therapist. On the other hand, the therapist, who had otherwise been committed to treating adolescents, says that, in fact, she wants to get rid of her, and that the patient should finally grow up. When asked what had triggered her negative countertransference, she spontaneously answers, visibly annoyed, that she did not want to be the patient's washing machine! In the further course, it turns out that the patient had been a cry-baby that could be calmed down only if the (annoyed) mother put her on the rotating washing machine. The mother had clearly failed to calm the patient as a baby using only her voice, prosody, or rhythmic movements; the washing machine seems to have been more successful in this regard. Once the analyst had processed the fact that the negative countertransference represented a repetition of the rejecting mother could accept the patient's wish for the analyst to be a resonating body and not a washing machine.

Notes

1 Is it a coincidence that the 2021 Nobel Prize in Medicine went to two molecular biology sensory researchers who discovered specific receptors for temperature and touch in the body?
2 It is possible that this partly results from the climate crisis in the form of heat waves, floods, and forest fires, which has heightened the perception of increased risks for bodily stress in the form of anxiety and panic disorders ("eco-anxiety"), violence, aggression, and posttraumatic stress disorder.
3 I owe this reference to Teresa von Sommeruga Howard (NZL) from the GASI Forum.

References

Adolphs, R. (2003): Cognitive neuroscience of human social behaviour. *Nat Rev Neurosci*, 4(3), 165–178.

Arbeitskreis-OPD (2014): *OPD 2 – Operationalisierte Psychodynamische Diagnostik: Das Manual für Diagnostik und Therapieplanung*. In: Opd, A. & Cierpka, M. (Eds.) 2nd ed. Bern: Huber.

Alexander, F. (1948): Fundamental concepts of psychosomatic research. Psychogenesis, conversion, specifity. *Psychosom Med*, 5, 205–210.

Anzieu, D. (2016 [1991]): *Das Haut-Ich*. Trans. by M. Korte u.M.-H. Lebourdais-Weiss. Frankfurt a.M.: Suhrkamp.

Bauer, J. (2005): *Warum Ich fühle, was Du fühlst. Intuitive Kommunikation und das Geheimnis der Spiegelneurone*. Hamburg: Hoffmann und Campe.

Beebe, B., Cohen, P. & Lachmann, F. (2019): *Bindung im Werden. Mikroanalyse der Mutter-Kind-Interaktion*. Gießen: Psychosozial.

Buchholz, M. B. (2003): *Neue Assoziationen. Psychoanalytische Lockerungsübungen*. Gießen: Psychosozial.

Buchholz, M. B. (2020): Seeing the situational gestalt – Movement in therapeutic spaces. *Gestalt Theory*, 42(2), 101–132.

Cardinal, M. (1979): *Schattenmund*. Reinbek: Rowohlt.

Deutsch, F. (1926): Der gesunde und der kranke Körper in psychoanalytischer Betrachtung. *Int Z Psychoanal*, 12(3), 493–503.

Di Cesare, G., Fasano, F., Errante, A., Marchi, M. & Rizzolatti, G. (2016): Understanding the internal states of others by listening to action verbs. *Neuropsychologia*, 89, 172–179. 10.1016/j.neuropsychologia.2016.06.017

Ehrenthal, J. C. (2019): Erfahrungsbasiertes Lernen psychodynamischer Interventionen. *Forum Psychoanal*, 35(4), 413–428.

Ferenczi, S. (1919): *Die Psychoanalyse der Kriegsneurosen. Internationale Psychoanalytische Bibliothek, Vol. 1*. Wien: Internationaler Psychoanalytischer Verlag, 9–30.

Ferenczi, S. (1919 [1984]): Hysterische Materialisationsvorgänge. Gedanken zur Auffassung der hysterischen Konversion und Symbolik. In: Ferenczi, S. (Ed.): *Bausteine zur Psychoanalyse*, Vol. III. Bern/Stuttgart/Wien: Huber, 3rd ed., 129–147.

Fonagy, P., Gergely, G., Jurist, E. L. & Target, M. (2002 [2004]): *Affect Regulation, Mentalization and the Development of the Self*. London/New York: Karnac.

Freud, S. (1913c) On Beginning the Treatment. SE XII, 121–144.

Freud, S. (1915c): Instincts and their Vicissitudes. SE XIV, 109–140.

Gaddini, E. (1998 [1981]): Bemerkungen zum Psyche-Soma-Problem. In: Gaddini, E.: *"Das Ich ist vor allem ein Körperliches." Beiträge zur Psychoanalyse der ersten Strukturen*. Jappe, G. & Strehlow, B. (Eds.). Frankfurt a. M.: Brandes & Apsel (edition diskord). 2nd ed., 21–51. 3rd exp. and corr. ed. 2016.

Henningsen, P. (2021): *Allgemeine Psychosomatische Medizin. Krankheiten des verkörperten Selbst im 21. Jahrhundert*. Heidelberg: Springer.

Isen, A. M., Daubman, K. A. & Nowicki, G. P. (1987): Positive affect facilitates creative problem solving. *Journal of Personality and Social Psychology*, 52, 1122–1131.

Karacaöğlan, U. (2012): Tattoo and taboo: On the meaning of tattoos in the analytic process. *Int J Psychoanal*, 93(1), 5–28.

Krause, R. (1992): Die Zweierbeziehung als Grundlage der psychoanalytischen Therapie. *Psyche – Z Psychoanal*, 46, 588–612.

Krause, R. (2016): Auf der Suche nach dem »missing link« zwischen Analytiker und Analysand, ihren Körpern und ihrer gemeinsamen Seele. Oder wie ist der intersubjektive Raum konstruiert und tapeziert? In: Nohr, K. & Leikert, S. (Eds.): *Zum Phänomen der Rührung in Psychoanalyse und Musik – Eine Publikation der Deutschen Gesellschaft für Psychoanalyse und Musik*. Gießen: Psychosozial.

Krause, S., Boeck, C., Gumpp, A. M., et al. (2018): Child maltreatment is associated with a reduction of the oxytocin receptor in peripheral blood mononuclear cells. *Front Psychol*, 9, 173.

Kuchuck, S. (2013): *Clinical Implications of the Psychoanalyst's Life Experience – When the Personal Becomes Professional*. London: Routledge.

Leikert, S. (2019): *Das sinnliche Selbst: Körpergedächtnis und psychoanalytische Behandlungstechnik*. Frankfurt a.M.: Brandes & Apsel.

Leikert, S. (2021): Encapsulated body engrams and somatic narration – Integrating body memory into psychoanalytic technique. *IJP*, 102(4), 671–688. 10.1080/002075 78.2021.1927044

Lemma, A. (2014): *Minding the body. The body in psychoanalysis and beyond*. London: Routledge. German

Lemma, A. (2018): *Der Körper spricht immer. Körperlichkeit in psychoanalytischen Therapien und jenseits der Couch*. Trans. by L. Apsel. Frankfurt a. M.: Brandes & Apsel.

Levy, J. & Feldman, R. (2019): Synchronous Interactions Foster Empathy. *J Exp Neurosci*, 13(1–2). 10.1177/1179069519865799

Lingiardi, V. & dei Bei, F. (2011): Questioning the couch: Historical and clinical perspectives. *Psychoanal Psychol*, 28, 389–404.

Lombardi, R. (2008): The body in the analytic session: Focusing on the body-mind link. *Int J Psychanal*, 89, 89–109.

Lombardi, R. (2017): *Body-mind dissociation in psychoanalysis: Development after Bion*. London/New York: Routledge. German

Ludwig-Körner, C. (2015): Und wer denkt an das Baby? Überlegungen zur Methode der Säuglingsbeobachtung. *Psyche – Z Psychoanal*, 69(12), 1162–1184.

Lynch, T. R., Rosenthal, M. Z., Kosson, D. S., Cheavens, J. S., Lejuez, C. W. & Blair, R. J. R. (2006): Heightened sensitivity to facial expressions of emotion in borderline personality disorder. *Emotion*, 6(4), 647–655.

Maier, A., Gieling, C., Heinen-Ludwig, L., Stefan, V., Schultz, J., Gunturkun, O., et al. (2020): Association of childhood maltreatment with interpersonal distance and social touch preferences in adulthood. *Am J Psychiatry*, 177(1), 37–46.

McDougall, J. (1991): *Theater des Körpers. Ein psychoanalytischer Ansatz für die psychosomatische Erkrankung*. Stuttgart: Internationale Psychoanalyse.

Merleau-Ponty, M. (1974 [1965]): *Phänomenologie der Wahrnehmung*. Berlin: de Gruyter.

Pankow, G. W. (1974): The body image in hysterical psychosis. *Int J Psychoanal*, 55, 407–414.

Panksepp, J. (2009): Brain emotional systems and qualities of mental life. From animal models of affect to implications for psychotherapeutics. In: Fosha, D., Siegel, D. J. & Solomon, M. F. (Eds.): *The Healing Power of Emotion. Affective Neuroscience, Development & Clinical Practice*. New York/London: Norton, 1–26.

Panksepp, J. & Biven, L. (2012): *The Archaeology of Mind. Neuroevolutionary Origins of Human Emotions*. New York/London: Norton.

Penfield, W. & Faulk, M. E., Jr. (1955): The insula: Further observations on its function. *Brain*, 78(4), 445–470.

Pflichthofer, D. (2008): *Spielräume des Erlebens. Performanz und Verwandlung in der Psychoanalyse*. Gießen: Psychosozial.

Plassmann, R. (1993): Organwelten: Grundriß einer analytischen Körperpsychologie. *Psyche – Z Psychoanal*, 47, 261–282.

Plassmann, R. (2019): *Psychotherapie der Emotionen. Die Bedeutung von Emotionen für die Entstehung und Behandlung von Krankheiten*. Gießen: Psychosozial.

Quinodoz, D. (2003): Words that touch. *Int J Psychoanal*, 84, 1469–1485.

Quinodoz, D. (2011): *Worte, die berühren. Eine Psychoanalytikerin lernt sprechen*. Frankfurt a. M.: Brandes & Apsel, 3rd ed.

Rizzolatti, G. & Sinigaglia, C. (2016): The mirror mechanism: A basic principle of brain function. *Nat Rev Neurosci*, 17(12), 757–765.

Rizzolatti, G., Fadiga, L., Fogassi, L. & Gallese, V. (1999): Resonance behaviors and mirror neurons. *Arch Ital Biol*, 137, 83–99.

Sandler, J. & Sandler, A. M. (1984): Vergangenheits-Unbewußtes, Gegenwarts-Unbewußtes und die Deutung der Übertragung. *Psyche – Z Psychoanal*, 39(9), 800–829.

Sato, W., Uono, S., Matsuura, N. & Toichi, M. (2009): Misrecognition of facial expressions in delinquents. *Child Adolesc Psychiatry Ment Health*, 3(1), 27.

Schachter, D. L. & Kächele, H. (2010): The couch in psychoanalysis. *Contemp Psychoanal*, 46, 439–459.

Scharff, J. M. (2010): *Die leibliche Dimension in der Psychoanalyse*. Frankfurt a. M.: Brandes & Apsel.

Scharff, J. M. (2021): *Psychoanalyse und Zwischenleiblichkeit. Klinisch-propädeutisches Seminar*. Frankfurt a. M.: Brandes & Apsel.

Schilder, P. (1978 [1935]): *The image and the appearance of the human body*. New York: International UP.

Schiller, B.-M. (2021). A case of trichotillomania and trichophagy: Fantasies of cannibalism. *Int J Psychoanal*, 1–21.

Schmidt, D. (2019): Zur therapeutischen Wirksamkeit von Handlungen in der Psychoanalyse. *Forum Psychoanal*, 3.

Schmidt, M. G. (2020): Zur therapeutischen Wirksamkeit von Handlungen in der Psychoanalyse. *Forum Psychoanal*, 36(3), 261–276.

Schröter, M. (2018): Die Psychoanalyse und die "Kriegsneurosen" des Ersten Weltkriegs – Eine zweideutige Probe aufs Exempel. *Psyche – Z Psychoanal*, 72, 122–145.

Schultz-Venrath, U. (1995 [1992]): *Ernst Simmels Psychoanalytische Klinik "Sanatorium Schloß Tegel GmbH" (1927–1931) – Beitrag zur Wissenschaftsgeschichte einer psychoanalytischen Psychosomatik*. Universität Witten/Herdecke 1992. Deutsche Hochschulschriften 2081, Mikroedition. Hänsel-Hohenhausen, Egelsbach, Frankfurt am Main, Washington.

Schultz-Venrath, U. (2015 [2013]): *Lehrbuch Mentalisieren. Psychotherapien wirksam gestalten*. Stuttgart: Klett-Cotta.

Schultz-Venrath, U. (2021): *Mentalisieren des Körpers*. Stuttgart: Klett-Cotta.

Schultz-Venrath, U. & Hermanns, L. M. (2019): Ernst Simmel oder die Psycho-Klinik der Zukunft. In: Geisthövel, A. & Hitzer, B. (Eds.): *Auf der Suche nach einer anderen Medizin – Psychosomatik im 20. Jahrhundert*. Frankfurt a. M.: Suhrkamp Taschenbuch Wissenschaft, 124–132.

Schwartz, M. A. & Wiggins, O. P. (1987): Typifications: The first step for clinical diagnosis in psychiatry. *J Nerv Ment Dis*, 175, 65–77.

Simmel, E. (1918): *Kriegsneurosen und »Psychisches Trauma«. Ihre gegenseitigen Beziehungen dargestellt auf Grund psycho-analytischer, hypnotischer Studien*. Leipzig München: Otto Nemnich.

Simmel, E. (1924): Die psycho-physische Bedeutsamkeit des Intestinalorgans für die Urverdrängung. *Int Z Psychoanal*, 10, 218–221.

Solms, M. (2021): *The Hidden Spring – A Journey to the Source of Consciousness*. New York: Norton.

Stegmann, M. (1926): Die Psychogenese organischer Krankheiten und das Weltbild. *Imago*, 12, 196–202.

Storck, T. (2021): Analysierte Körper. In: Wilm, H., Unterthurner, G., Storck, T., Kadi, U. & Boelderl, A. S. (Eds.): *Körperglossar*. Wien/Berlin: Turia + Kant, 13–17.

Storebo, O. J., Stoffers-Winterling, J. M., Vollm, B. A., Kongerslev, M. T., Mattivi, J. T., Jorgensen, M. S., et al. (2020): Psychological therapies for people with borderline personality disorder. *Cochrane Database Syst Rev*, 5(5), CD012955. 10.1002/14651858. CD012955.pub2

Strzelczyk, A. & Schmitt, F. C. (2020): 100 Jahre Dieter Janz. *Zeitschrift für Epileptologie*, 33, 101–106.

Trevarthen, C. (1979): Communication and cooperation in early infancy: A description of primary intersubjectivity. In: Bullowa, M. (Ed.): *Before Speech: The Beginning of Interpersonal Communication.* Cambridge, UK: Cambridge University Press, 321–347.

Trevarthen, C. & Aitken, K. J. (2001): Infant intersubjectivity: Research, theory, and clinical applications. *J Child Psychol Psychiatry*, 42(1), 3–48.

Varela, F., Thompson, E. & Rosch, E. (2016 [1991]): *The Embodied Mind.* Cambridge, MA: MIT.

Volz-Boers, U. (2001): Mit Leib und Seele: Körpererfahrungen und subsymbolische Kommunikation in der Gegenübertragung. In: Schlösser, A.-M. & Gerlach, A. (Eds.): *Kreativität und Scheitern.* Gießen: Psychosozial, 385–396.

Volz-Boers, U. (2004): Facetten des Unbewußten: Unbewußtes und Körperempfindungen in der Gegenübertragung. In: Ardjomandi, M. E. (Ed.): *Jahrbuch für Gruppenanalyse und ihre Anwendungen – Trennung, Trauer und Aufbruch in Gruppen,* Vol. 10. Weimar: Mattes, 155–167.

Volz-Boers, U. (2007): Psychoanalyse mit Leib und Seele. Körperliche Gegenübertragung als Zugang zu nicht symbolisierter Erfahrung und neuer Repräsentanzenbildung. In: Geißler, P. & Heisterkamp, G. (Eds.): *Psychoanalyse der Lebensbewegungen. Zum körperlichen Geschehen in der psychoanalytischen Therapie. Ein Lehrbuch.* Berlin: Springer, 39–58.

Volz-Boers, U. (2009): Körperempfindungen des Analytikers als Zugang zu perinataler Traumatisierung. In: Ardjomandi, M. E. (Ed.): *Jahrbuch für Gruppenanalyse und ihre Anwendungen – Wohin mit der Gruppenanalyse?* Vol. 14. Weimar: Mattes, 159–169.

Watt, D. F. (2017): Reflections on the neuroscientific legacy of Jaak Panksepp (1943–2017). *Neuropsychoanalysis*, 19(2), 183–198.

Wegner, P. & Henseler, H. (1991): Die Anfangsszene des Erstinterviews im Prisma einer Analytikergruppe. *Forum Psychoanal*, 7, 214–224.

v. Weizsäcker, V. (1954): Natur und Geist. Erinnerungen eines Arztes. In: Achilles, P., Janz, D., Schrenck, M. & von Weizsäcker, C. F. (Eds.): *Gesammelte Schriften 1.* Frankfurt a. M.: Suhrkamp, 9–189.

Chapter 9

Corporeality and Dream-Talk

Ewa Kobylinska-Dehe

Introduction

We learn from our patients. They take us off the beaten path to silent experiences that wish to be expressed. A unique language is developed along these tangled paths, a language used to communicate with only one particular patient.

For a long time, I failed to see, how tense and stiff Marie was, as she lay on the couch, giving off a smell I tried to ignore. I initially failed to notice that Paul would march to the couch in a decisive manner. He was sweaty and in tears upon finally reaching it. Anne would mumble less and less articulately, barely breathing, and finally fall silent as the grave. Adrian liked to doze off on the couch and dream. I enjoyed watching his rhythmic breathing and would let my eyes wander toward the trees whose leaves moved following a similar rhythm.

As my attention toward my patient´s sensory expression grew, I started to see, hear, and feel what was going on in a much more comprehensive and responsive manner. In this regard, I asked myself: How to find a language capable of doing justice to this sensual spectrum. A language that would not only replace old meanings with new ones, but rather a language that is effective and transformative. One that Bion dreamt of, inspired by the great English poet John Keats.

Every psychoanalyst faces the following challenge: **How to let experiences speak for themselves instead of speaking about them, as is often the case.** My patients were the ones who guided me toward a sensory dream-talk that we created together.

Marie said: "I feel my body dancing on a tightrope today." To which I replied: "From being stiff to tightrope dancing – that's a looong way to go." I inadvertently stretched the "o" sound in the word "long." I later realized that I had tried to emphasize the movement, rather than the possibility of losing balance or the omnipotent fantasy.

Paul saw himself as a marching soldier. At some point I said: "A courageous soldier with a weeping soul. Today, you are sad as only children

DOI: 10.4324/9781003370130-9

can be." Paul turned into a child for a moment. He repeated the word "courageous" by separating it into syllables and changing intonation each time: "coura-geous, cou-ra-ge-ous," and finally the short and decisive: "courageous!" Was he starting to play with me?

After returning to my office following a long absence caused by the pandemic, Marie stared at a bunch of flowers.

She asked:	"Are these real?"
A:	"As real as you and me."
P:	"May I touch them?"
A:	"Of course. They don't bite."
P:	(serious but with a slightly mischievous smile): "What if they do?"

Then, she touched one of the leaves cautiously and stated contentedly: "They're real."

This way, we "worked through" the first meeting in the office after a break. The session was filled with an array of emotional meanings than no discursive-verbal interpretation was capable of containing and expressing: closeness, distance, touch, fear, authenticity, seriousness, play, joy, and caution.

Of course, therapeutic sessions are not just about these, as I call them, **poetic moments**. But if the muse is kind, these moments appear, and they are essential for transformation processes. A poetic moment allows us to remain in the openness of the mind. A successful analytic session is, following Loewald, "an artistic creation fashioned by patient and analyst in collaboration. [...] The progression in such an hour is quite similar to the progression of a work of art, a poem, a musical composition" (Loewald, 1975, pp. 296–297).

My chapter will focus on the issue of mediating between the body and the mind. I will argue that dream-talk, as the primary expression, is the missing link between the bodily and the mental. It transforms the biological body into a bodily self, which allows a non-possessive cathexis of our own body. To feel alive in the world one has to first feel alive in one's own body.

German sociologist Ulrich Oevermann uses the notion of **bodily positioning** to describe the core of the individual sense of being alive, which cannot be fully captured in physical, biological, mental, or cultural terms. It constitutes the nucleus of human subjectivity and the point of departure for future processes of development and individualization. In consequence, what is given is transformed into a unique individual project. Winnicott describes the process of coming into being in a similar manner. In his theory, a "transitional object" and a "transitional space" serve as a kind of bridge between infant and mother and, at the same time, between the external and the internal in the separation process. These two very different authors both express an intuition that human beings have to accept what is given and transform it into a unique project of themselves, continually exceeding the self. It is the only way one can settle comfortably in one's body as a subject and, still, never feel fully at home. Let us now examine this process, its disruptions, and how it is addressed in clinical situations.

How Does a Biological Body Become a Bodily Experience?

In the beginning, before a narrative form develops, we are immersed in a chaotic universe of stimuli, sounds, noises, smells, touches, and movements. For a body to become endowed with subjectivity, disorganized sensory impressions have to accepted, dreamed, and, in consequence, integrated. Every mother addresses her baby as an individual, a "you." She calls it by its name and dreams about it, instead of just satisfying its biological needs.

We may now start a theoretical deliberation on how the innate disposition to develop pre-symbolic categories and to imitate, discovered by researchers who had studied infants, and the idea that perception, as an organizing, forming, and communicating activity from the very beginning, are compatible with the concepts of proto-emotive chaos and incoherent masses of unprocessed stimuli formulated by Bion and his followers. However, in clinical practice it is irrelevant whether we are dealing with a primary state or whether this state develops as a result of disturbance, such as traumatic separation, mother's inability to reverie, or child's hypersensitivity. Either way, in such clinical cases, transition from pure sensations to experiencing them emotionally, expressing with words, and finally understanding them seems unbridgeable. In these cases, self-communication and the bodily core of existence are separated. Lombardi notices that such a deep body–mind separation differs from both hysterical dissociation (Freud) and schizoid mechanism (Klein). They are both concerned with the modes of processing emotions that have already been shaped into an elementary mental organization (Lombardi, 2016, p. 78). Differently, the disconnection discussed here goes deeper, to the level of the elementary attunement of body to mind and mind to body. We might say, from a philosophical point of view, that such patients are the children of Descartes.

From the viewpoint of phenomenology, the question of embodying a biological body is posed incorrectly. Only in Descartes's philosophical tradition, a physical body (*res extensa*) is seen as a polar opposite of psyche (*res cogitans*). In everyday life, the two artificially separated spheres are closely linked.

The Paris Psychosomatic School draws on the phenomenological tradition much more than the British or German schools (Storck & Brauner, 2021, p. 36). Marty, de M'uzan, or McDougall all believe that a non-pathological process is characterized by a constant exchange between soma, psyche, and the environment. This dynamic interpenetration resembles Merleau-Ponty's concept of "intercorporeity." However, this process may be disrupted. From this viewpoint, operatory thinking (*pensée operatoire*) or alexithymia signify a dissociation from affective-bodily processes rather than deficits in mentalization (Fonagy). Hence, psychosomatic disturbances result from drive pathology and, to use Winnicott's words, from a disturbance of the sense of being alive.

Thomas Ogden described the experience of elementary mental expression as an autistic-contiguous position and was the first to focus on it in clinical work. It is typically believed that Freud did not find access to this fundamental experience. However, as Loewald claims, psychoanalysis would not have been established without Freud's particular interest in body signals. For Loewald, Freud's drives are not purely biological impulses or abstract constructs, but the life of the body:

> kisses and excrements [...], tastes and smells and sights, body noises and sensations, caresses and punishments, tics and gait and movements [...], pain and pleasure, physical excitement and lassitude, violence and bliss – all this is the body in the context of human life. (Loewald, 1971, p. 114)

Drives as psychic forces come to being from the field of mother–infant interaction. Infant's uncoordinated movements, its breathing, digesting, or crying does not yet have the nature of a drive, nor it is a mental representation. Only as a result of motherly responses, kinesthetic patterns are developed that, in turn, create the drives (cf. Loewald, 1971, p. 120). While a biological body exists, a bodily self has to come into being. The first sensory experiences are both stimulated and modulated by the maternal reverie. The latter is not simply nonverbal. The mother speaks.

Loewald's reinterpretation of Freud's theory of drives deserves attention because, while he still positions it in the center of the psychoanalytic theory of the body, he adds a component of relation and mediation. A "drive" is an excess of body stimuli that forces creation of representations. Let us complete Loewald's concept with Bernhard Waldenfels's reinterpretation of the drive theory. This philosopher and phenomenologist perceives the drives' dynamic as a game of pathos and response. A thing does not just appear in our sight when we intentionally direct our attention to "it." "It" appears to us when it touches us and affects us. This "thing" is not only a biological stimulus with a measurable intensity. It is a demand that requires a response and not simply a reaction. Representation becomes a response. It is therefore not a question of stimuli but of pathic moments, enigmatic messages from the other, who deserves our response. The dynamic of pathos and response clearly demonstrates the difference between a drive and an instinct.

In conclusion to this part of my chapter, I will say that, first, Freud's concept of the body was close to our current psychoanalytic understanding of it.

Additionally, he did recognize the creative process of transformation of a biological body into a libidinal–phantasmatic body by means of motherly responses, cathexis, and stimulations. Finally, he knew how to exploit the sensuality and visuality of the (German) language.

Let us digress for a moment: French writer, Georges-Arthur Goldschmidt, in his wonderful book, *Quand Freud voit la mer* (When Freud Sees the Sea), attempted to understand psychoanalysis from the viewpoint of Freud's usage of language. He reached a surprising conclusion that almost no other language is as bodily as Freud's German. In contrast to the French language, "many German words make what they describe, visual, sensual, and almost physically tangible" (Goldschmidt, 2006, p. 41). *Krankenwagen* (ambulance) is *wagen* (car) transporting *Kranken* (the ill); *Krankenhaus* (hospital) is *Haus* (house) for the ill. Something is *unheimlich* (uncanny) because it visits us in our own *Heim* (home). When I talk with my German patients, I sometimes hear something that a native speaker would miss, as a result of the process of conventionalization of semantics. In *Über-ich* (Superego), I immediately see someone standing on my shoulders (lit. *Über* = over, above; *Ich* = me). When I hear the word *Mariahimmelfahrt* (the Assumption of Virgin Mary), I smile because I picture Mary getting into a taxi and driving to heaven (heaven: *Himmel*; *Fahrt* = trip). In the "responsibility" (*Verantwortung*), I hear "response." In the word *Trieb* (drive), I immediately hear an entire list of words: *Trieb* (sprout), *treiben* (to rush), *treiben* (to pursue), *Treibholz* (driftwood), *Treibsand* (quicksand), etc. Also in more abstract expressions, such as *Sachverhalt* (state of affairs, matters), I immediately see how *Sache* (the affairs) behave (*Verhalten* = behavior). In *Wesensschau*, I look directly at *Wesen* (the essence). In the word *Leib* (body), I hear *Leben* (life). Goldschmidt emphasizes the material aspect of key Freudian terms, which derive meanings simply from being "gestural, figurative, and close to spoken, everyday language" (Goldschmidt, 2006, p. 42). Freud did not change the semantic fields but rather exploited (exhausted) them. The vibrancy of his language enabled him to "explore the sensory experience of life as well as the material and bodily relationship to space" (Goldschmidt, 2006, p. 50). Even if Freud did not have a lot in common with the maternal *lalangue* (Lacan), he did have an unwavering sense of the bodily, figurative character of the German language, and he never surpassed it by creating artificial constructs.

We are currently observing a certain convergence between the philosophical phenomenology of the body, embodied cognitive science, and modern psychoanalysis. Bion, Ogden, Anzieu, and Lombardi all underline the importance of the body in both the functions of mind and the development of object relations. The processing of dreams and the bodily reality are pivotal in these processes, which may still be interrupted. Thus, a psychoanalytic process should not be limited to an exploration of fantasies. It should enable patients to experience, in their bodies, "the mysterious psychosensorial experience of being ourselves" (Lombardi, 2016, p. 93).

My exceptionally intelligent patient, Marie, used abstract vocabulary characteristic for her professional field, but was incapable of experiencing emotions. I, on the other hand, under the power of projective identification, was unable to be spontaneous and "forgot" about my body. We both kept on freezing motionlessly. Once, as if from afar, I heard a quiet calling: "Please, say something, so that I can feel my body." I felt so paralyzed inside that nothing came to my mind. I began to move restlessly. My body reminded me of itself. I told Marie about it. "This is exactly the state I am in," she replied and started moving her legs slowly. I was astonished; the words of the Freudian child came to my mind: "if anyone speaks, it gets light" (Freud, 1905d, p. 224). Bodily experiences cannot be separated into individual sensory channels (including the speaking channel). Marie needed to hear my voice to reclaim the sensations pertaining to her own body and to be able to move her feet. The embodied subjectivity, constitutive to a human being, allows us to feel, express ourselves, speak, and act with our entire bodies (cf. Fuchs, 2021, p. 36).

Time and Space of the Body

Bion radically reconceptualized Freud's ideas. Instead of focusing on the repressed content and defense mechanisms, he addressed the patterns of mental functioning and the disruptions of psyche in connection to the body. Ogden went a step further than Bion. He argued that sense of being alive in one's body constitutes the core of the self, the point of reference to the universe, and the beginning of differentiated thinking.

The tridimensionality of the body as the primary "container" is the precondition for the establishment of a bodily time-space. The latter limits the flood of emotional states and is essential for creating representations. However, this tridimensionality remains in constant tension with the human tendency to transgress into infinity. As a result, archaic states occur as pure sensations beyond time and space. Referring to Freudian distinction between primary and secondary processes, Lombardi points toward two organizations: symmetrical and asymmetrical. The former blurs the differences and boundaries. The latter simultaneously differentiates and limits. Contrary to Freud, but similarly to Bion and Ogden, Lombardi emphasizes the continuous oscillation of the two "logics" between the finite and the infinite.

The parameters of space and time play a cornerstone role in every analysis because they organize bodily sensations. Marie did not initially understand the term "space." She would ask: "What are you trying to tell me?" or "What do you mean?" Only when she began to experience space by walking around the office, she was able to feel it and to develop preconceptions. Only then, she was able to name her feelings. She would say, for example, that she has gained more space or that she is feeling more confined. Previously, she had lacked the words to express this.

During Marie's analysis, I noticed that she, or both of us, would occasionally perform a concrete action that also had a symbolic dimension.

At the beginning of one of our sessions, she asked me: "What are we going to do today?" and I replied spontaneously: "How about we go for a walk?"

Marie: "Metaphorical or a literal one?"
Analyst: "Both?"
M: "Do you mean that I'm moving during the session? ... But I can't really move around or go for a walk here?"
A: "Why not?"
M: "Ok, I'll do it."

She got up, carefully approached the window, raising her knees high like a stork, and then sat down again, saying, "funny." It was a bodily experience beyond both the objectivist understanding of a body and the pure meaning of words. Some years later, Marie revealed to me that the process of creating mental space in connection to bodily sensations was for her the most important experience during analysis.

To use Lombardi's notion, the experience of her own body allowed her to emerge from the **formless infinity**. A tridimensional body organizes space and time. In each position: lying down, sitting up, or walking, we experience space differently. The human body does not only move in space. It also configures space and shapes it, and in doing so, it establishes a reference to the world. Hence, our perception depends on our physical position. When Marie laid down on the couch, after two years of sitting opposite me, her new position changed her perception as well as mine. Our being together in the office became more tangible and sensual in this nonconventional situation, for example, at a time of bodily falling out of sync followed by an attempt at retuning. When she went to lay down for the first time, it turned out that my movements were not coordinated with hers. She has just sat on the couch, while I had already been in a relaxed, reclined position in my armchair. When I noticed the discrepancy, I corrected my posture, but Marie was already laying down stiff like a board. We were out of step. I smelled fear. I synchronized with her rapid breathing, and the rhythm slowed down. Her feet slightly turned in a childlike way. I leaned my head in closer because she spoke very quietly. We converged cautiously. "From the couch, the world looks different ... somehow more coherent." Marie initiated a mental game: "One is more with oneself, and when you sit where I can gaze at you briefly, I feel your presence."

Apart from space, the category of time played an important role in this process. Toward the end of our sessions, Marie would start panicking: "We are out of time ... everything is spinning in my head faster and faster ... exploding ... I have so many thoughts at once. That's why I can't talk." Alternatively, to these catastrophes, she would feel locked in a timeless state. I tried simple timely interventions: "slowly, one thing at a time," etc. The experience of introducing spatial and time limits with Marie was remarkable.

Words like: "a little," "step by step," "earlier," and "later" became important messages in our communication. Marie, who lived in constant anxiety and tension due to disorientation, a state of paralysis, breakdowns, and a flood of emotions, started to create boundaries. She once said: "I need a moment, I'm just getting ready." She began to think: "I can describe here the state I am in. But you have to use a quiet voice."

Based on this foundation, a sense of a phantasmatic dimension of temporality started to develop – one that was previously unknown to Marie. What I understand by it is the movement of hesitation, anticipation, foreboding, returning, and renewing. Additionally, a multidimensional experience of time, the multiple layers of time coexisting in one person.

Gradually, Marie gained the capacity of letting her thoughts come and go freely instead of just having or not having thoughts. The route led from a pure sensory experience, through experiencing feelings, to primary expression associated with sensual activity, and finally to thinking. By differentiating elementary sensory experiences, my patient started to distinguish between different emotions. Everyday emotional contact was not evoking the feelings of confusion and intolerable excitement in her anymore – frequently experienced in the past. For a while, Marie preferred to talk over the phone, to be able to regulate and differentiate the influx of stimuli. In the office, she was incapable of sharing physical space with me while being in touch with herself and with me. One of us would always disappear. Either she took possession of me or perceived my presence as an intrusion on her sphere. Overwhelmed with intolerable states, she was only being able to scream: "too much, too much!" She aptly called this state, the collapse of space. She defended herself against the deluge with highly abstract constructs. In the end, she was either submerged or heavily armored.

Marie's communications often resembled explosions. She was trying to contain so much that it would blow up the container. Words were supposed to provide shapes for feelings, but would instead disintegrate into nonarticulated particles. Because of explosions, there was no space for images to emerge, and therefore the particles took on a persecutory character.

Initially, Marie undermined all my attempts at creating space because she perceived them as intrusive. Her states persecuted and terrified her. She grappled with her body. At times, her entire body was in pain; other times, she could not feel it at all. Occasionally, the most basic words would cause a shift, for example, when I said: "A tear is coursing down your cheek." Sometimes, rarely, at the end of a session, a subtle feeling, fragile like a flower would appear: "Thank you for listening," she whispered once as she was leaving.

During the period of telephone communications, Marie discovered that it was easier for her to be in touch with herself in the space of her own apartment. When she returned to my office 3 months later, she seemed more delimited. She stopped checking if the doors and windows in her apartment were closed. The new boundaries enabled Marie to create space in which she could experience emotions. She began to express them with poetic images. I repeated them to emphasize their strength. It was dream-talk that bridged sensory hypersensitivity with high-level abstraction. The abstract constructs had separated Marie from hypersensitivity to bodily sensations. At the same time, they had provided a type of a protective container. Marie: "I am capable of talking about everything but I am completely out of touch with myself. When I try to feel myself at least a little, it suddenly becomes a lot, it is about to explode, and I get so blocked that I cannot speak at all." Only the images, which I perceived as poetic and created by Marie, would ease the split slightly and enable Marie to start a conversation between her body and mind. It is essential that an analyst does not interrupt this process and remains in the background. In the spirit of Winnicott's **environmental mother**, I supported my patient's dialog with her bodily experiences and held off with offering my interpretation of transference. The first stage was the development of a mental structure; interpretation was the second.

When the patient developed mental space and became anchored in her body, she was able to cautiously open up to personal relations (Lombardi). Previously, she had paralyzed and silenced me. I was not allowed to have my own gestures or words. "Don't interrupt me," she would cut me off each time, even when all I said was "mm-hmm" or when I took a deeper breath. It took me a long time to realize that her "no" was not only denial but even rejection. It represented a desperate attempt to establish her own boundaries necessary to enter a relationship. Marie's boundaries had been continuously violated. As a result, she was incapable of feeling them and internalizing them, which is a necessary condition for developing a representation of the body and the self.

From Reverie to Dream-Talk

Bion's reverie differs from Freud's concept of evenly suspended attention. While the latter focused on methodical suspension of presuppositions allowing to notice something new, Bion understood it is an aura, a distant intimacy, which allows for a fluidity of things and has a healing effect. While Bion predominantly described reverie as maternal receptivity toward her child's projective identification, Ogden expanded this concept by describing an entire array of states affecting an analyst, including their physical state. He framed the concept as an experience that is both personal and intersubjective. But how to "translate" the capacity for reverie, understood as an attitude or state, into speaking or even interpretation? How can maternal reverie, which includes nursing, rocking, caressing, lulling, humming, and talking, be found in analysis?

Reverie has both the bodily and the speaking quality. Maternal reverie is always connected with a voice and communication that transforms the biological body into subjective corporeality. This experience taints us for life and shapes our physicality: How we move, how we talk, and even our sexual styles. This is simultaneously an experiencing body and an experienced body, which interacts with itself and others, anchored in the lifeworld (*Lebenswelt*) and carrying traces of past relations. On the primary level, this experience precedes the distinction between "I" and "you" and before the mechanisms of projection and introjection are at work, which imply a fundamental separateness (Lombardi).

Voice connects the body with language. We unknowingly use many different voices with our patients: calming, reserved, patient, or emotional (Ogden). Our patients also speak in many different tones of voice. Some complain or moan; others have a haunting voice. Some, on the contrary, have a deep voice that is so melodic that one would like to listen to it for a long time, but this voice does not match the patient's childish behavior. Others constantly interrupts themselves with laughter or just fall silent mid-sentence. Especially, "early-disturbed" patients listen closely to the sound of their analyst's voice. One of them told me: "Your voice is hard. And now, it is soft again." The "fingerprint quality of the voice" (Dolar) assigns it individuality but, contrary to a fingerprint, it cannot be identified once and for all. Therefore, the voice sustains "an intimate link with the very notion of the subject" and the other (Dolar, 2006, p. 23). It is simultaneously a presence and a disappearance. It can be heard here and now, but it does not stay and cannot be kept. Reverie shares this ephemerality. They both carry a session and then disappear. Traces they leave behind cannot be pinned down with an unambiguous word.

Meaning is also carried by the tone of voice. To put it differently, meaning cannot be clearly separated from timbre, reverberation, echo, resonance, and pitch (cf. Dolar, 2006, p. 22). Lacan was initially inspired by de Saussure's structural linguistics, where phonemes lack sound substance. Then, the French psychoanalyst turned his attention away from *linguisterie* or linguistics toward *lalangue*. The latter is not language understood as a chain of signifiers nor a language understood only in terms of sounds. These are "points of convergence, of crosscuts, intersections, where the sound conflation functions as the break of signification and at the same time the source of another signification" (Dolar, 2006, p. 144). Hence, voice and meaning cannot be strictly opposed. The system of differences cannot grasp the subtle gradations of sound. There are no gaps between signifiers but rather a common texture. Therefore, Merleau-Ponty's point of departure was not a system but a linguistic environment (*milieu*). It is an element (*La chair, la mère*, the flesh, the mother) and a formative environment for speakers (cf. Merleau-Ponty, 2012, p. 185). Signifiers and signified interpenetrate. Expression is a combination of what was articulated and what was left unsaid. Therefore, semiotics of dream-talk cannot exist. Intonation or timbre do not disappear in signifiers without a trace. In this context, speaking is a bodily gesture, and the existential meaning precedes the semantic meaning.

However, if that's the case, what about the difference or negativity that occupies an important place in modern psychoanalysis (a negation of psychoanalytic hermeneutics, the work of the negative). I would like to speak up for the non-appropriating positivity expressed in the dreamy, insatiable, bodily speaking, that precedes the negative. Indeed, the bodily and musical qualities of the voice allow us to experience primal pleasure before this experience is negativized. We need fullness before we are confronted with absence.

A prominent linguist, Roman Jakobson, eventually dropped the question, "how is meaning produced by sounds?" and returned to his favorite subject: poetics and the question, "how are poetic qualities produced in language?" For Jakobson, repetitions, rhythms, rhymes, and sounds constitute the power of poetry. Speaking is never just about ascribing meaning. There is always more happening on the way to the meaning: "The voice beyond words is a senseless play of sensuality, it possesses a dangerous attractive force, although in itself it is empty and frivolous" (Dolar, 2006, p. 43). Hence, the need for an aesthetic form, a poetics of the unconscious, that allows to channel this excess. Indeed, we know a lot about Freud's fear of the singing sirens:

> [W]orks of art o exercise a powerful effect on me. […] [W]ith music, I am almost incapable of obtaining any pleasure. Some […] analytic turn of min in me rebels against being moved by a thing without knowing why I am thus affected and what it is that affects me. (Freud, 1914c, p. 122)

Hence, both absence and excess may be the source of the alien experience in intercorporeity. It would be a misunderstanding to equate it with intersubjectivity. Not identicality, but rather *chiasmus*, the crossing and intertwining, causes our bodies to be permeated with alienness. However, it is not a question of semiotic negation or self-alienation. Paradoxically, the connection with oneself occurs through detachment from oneself. The former is not just a negative experience of absence, but also a positive experience of transgressing, being moved, and being awed. Simply speaking, it is an experience of reverie whose alienness takes the form of concern, astonishment, surprise, or openness to the unknown (cf. Kobylinska-Dehe, 2021, p. 45). It is dream-talk, with its gaps, interruptions, and insatiable meanings, that holds and carries us. In this sense, dream-talk is a process or an anticipation instead of a rushed identification. It assumes an interpenetration of thinking and dreaming. Waldenfels talks about the in-between realm of dialog, Ogden – about the talking-as-dreaming. Both have in mind an openness of experience that transcends what is given and cannot be encapsulated in a ready-made language. Dream-talk and dream-listening open a scene onto another scene by mapping some trajectories while leaving others to remain unmarked fields. Dream-talk fluidizes what is ready and closed while creating a kind of space for responding to traumatic shock.

One day, during a session, my therapist colleague was sitting by an open window overlooking the garden. A patient was tormenting her with projections. When she attacked her with yet another projection: "You just want me to take the meds," my colleague replied pensively: "I can hear the fox scream in the garden." This allowed her to leave the patient's projective discourse for a while. A patient fell silent and then remembered the fox from *The Little Prince*. Instead of offering a direct interpretation, my colleague introduced a new perspective and heard patient's suffering (her scream). If she had said been straightforwardly: "I hear your scream," it probably would have pushed the patient even further into projective delusions.

From the phrase "the fox screams in the garden" emerged a poetic image that touched something while maintaining the distance. A scream can turn into a call providing someone hears it.

> The first scream may be caused by pain, by the need for food, by frustration and anxiety, but the moment the other hears it, the moment it assumes the place of its addressee the moment the other is provoked and interpellated by it, the moment it responds to it, scream retroactively turns into appeal, it is interpreted, endowed with meaning, it is transformed into a speech addressed to the other. (Dolar, 2006, p. 27)

One of my patients, Aleksandra, had the tendency to jump between sobs that resembled a scream of a wounded animal and intellectual distance. One day she came to my office filled with doubt: "I am confused because I don't know what you mean to me, who you are to me. On the one hand, we are sometimes so close and yet so far apart, strangers distant." At a loss of words, I stammered: "Maybe we should ... be distant ... to be close." P: "With my mother it is the other way around. And it breaks my heart." Then, following a longer moment of silence, she asked: "Do you know Schumann's song 'The Prophet Bird'? It calls longingly. When we were silent just now, I hummed it quietly to myself and I felt lighter." Analyst: "I cannot sing a song for you but I can share with you Robert Frost's poem that had inspired me." In the poem, a woman's voice contributes new sounds to the song of the birds that impact the tone despite having no words:

> Admittedly an eloquence so soft
> Could only have had an influence on birds
> When call or laughter carried it aloft.
> Be that as may be, she was in their song.
> Moreover her voice upon their voices crossed
> Had now persisted in the woods so long
> That probably it would never be lost.
>
> Never again would birds' song be the same. (Frost, 1942, p. 394)

P: "I would like your voice to stay inside me ..." We both remained in reverie until the end of the session. First, the conversation, then her humming of Schumann, and finally the poem introduced a moment of reverie that calmed my patient. She became gentler. Maternal reverie is, above all, receiving and opening the space, in which a scream turns into a call that requires a response.

Merleau-Ponty pointed toward *la chose intersensorielle* or an intersensorial thing understood as a combination of senses:

If a phenomenon – such as a reflection or a light breeze – only presents itself to one my senses, then it is a phantom, and it will only approach real existence if, by luck, it becomes capable of speaking to my other senses, as when the wind, for example, is violent and makes itself visible in the disturbances of the landscape. (Merleau-Ponty, 2012, p. 332)

Reverie allows us to dream up or imagine a missing component. It becomes unrealistic or hyperreal on the computer screen or over the phone. Marie was faced with a dilemma. On the one hand, when we talked over the phone for several months, she was less exposed to external stimuli, and it was easier for her to be in touch with herself. On the other hand, since she was (yet) unable to dream and to hold me inside her, she needed to see me in person to physically confirm my existence.

Marie would react to the experience of motherlessness with a silent weep and numbing of her body. I shared with her Olga Tokarczuk's "reverie," with which she opened her Nobel Lecture. She describes a photograph of her mother:

The first photograph I ever experienced consciously is a picture of my mother from before she gave birth to me. [...] The woman is sad, seemingly lost in thought – seemingly lost. When I later asked her about that sadness – which I did on numerous occasions, always prompting the same response – my mother would say that she was sad because I hadn't been born yet, yet she already missed me. "How can you miss me when I'm not there yet?" I would ask. [...] [S]he answered [...] "Missing a person means they're there." (Tokarczuk, 2018)

Marie: "I never had a mother. I don't know how it feels to have a mother." It was painful to hear but, this time, Marie did not resort to panic. Instead, she vaguely remembered that she had once heard her mother sing beautifully. It was a different feeling to an earlier situation from two years ago: I had felt tired during a session and then suddenly heard her loud call: "Are you still there?!" To my inarticulate "mm-hmm," she had replied in a panicked voice: "Your body is here but you are not – and I cannot feel my own body." Only then I had realized the seriousness of the situation: a bodily self-loss. Even a brief distraction of her therapist resulted in a disorganization of Marie's corporeality she had been in the process of regaining. She went into an emergency mode; she couldn't breathe, experienced leg numbness, and failed to get up. I firmly intervened: "Place one leg in front of the other. Good, now you've got the ground." A combination of sensory intensification and lack of an object resulted in experiencing unpleasant sensory sensations as catastrophic. For that reason, Marie tended to exercise firm control over affects and her body that, in turn, cut her off from the emotional context.

In a similar situation during a later session, when Marie couldn't feel her feet, all it took was an encouragement to alternately swing her legs. My encouragement but, above all, her own self-agency before she was ready to enter a personal relationship with her analyst. Experiencing oneself in a bodily manner, by embodying, registering, and differentiating between reliable sensory experiences, creates preconditions for entering a profound relationship with another human being.

During one of our sessions, Marie told me about her all-embracing loneliness in an intense manner that evoked my need to console her. Marie: "I don't need this right now. For the first time in my life, I can feel that these weird and anxiety-triggering states that had accompanied me throughout my childhood, are sadness and loneliness. I can name them." Marie was becoming herself and gaining subjectivity, while I hastened to offer a relationship.

Sandra would react to her visual impairment (strabismus) that had been unrecognized by her attractive mother by avoiding eye contact and hiding her face under a messy hairstyle that made her look unattractive. I connected with her by smell. When I told her she smelled in a very nice way, she replied with a story about her unusual sensitivity to smells and fondness of scents. This confession enhanced her self-confidence and trust in herself. Only then I dared to acknowledge her visual defect, while Sandra gradually worked up the courage to reveal her face.

These are examples of micro-scenes shaped by voice, gaze, smell, or body position that open the path leading to the other. In some cases, I gained access to my patients by observing their most basic, everyday gestures: How they move, sit down, lay down, and get up. All of these gestures have a component of elementary symbolism because to perceive them is different from both observing what is objectively given and a purely mental activity. Perception establishes a relationship with the world. Our intentions take on a visible form of expression through our bodies. We may say that expression co-creates meaning, not just expresses it.

All phenomena occurring during a psychoanalytic session are messages: Responses and, at the same time, expressions of the patient's and analyst's subjectivity. There are many different forms of communication and emotional resonance, and many ways of expressing difficult experiences – even for one and the same patient. The process of working through involves not only talking and interpreting, but also scenes, dreams, moments of silence, symbolic actions, and dream-talk.

Concepts of body memory presume that elementary form of representation occurs even in the case of so-called unrepresented states – in fact, with the body. Everything that appears in the session is represented, but this representation does not have to always occur in a highly symbolic manner. Take the example of paralysis. If one experiences paralysis of a non-organic origin, one communicates that one perceives and feels what had happened to him as paralysis. Like the above-mentioned cry, paralysis turns into a message, a call directed at the analyst. The mental articulates itself in a bodily manner. In fact, sharp distinctions between represented and unrepresented states, bodily and psychic pain replicate established cartesian schemata and reduce our clinical possibilities.

To understand the role of the body in the process of activating memories, we must acknowledge that it goes beyond the constitutive awareness of the past. It is rather an effort to reopen time from the present viewpoint. The body allows us to experience space and time. Marcel Proust described it more accurately than scientists:

> For it always happened that when I like this, and my mind struggled in an unsuccessful attempt to discover where I was, everything revolved around me through the darkness: things, places, years. My body [...] [i]ts memory, the composite memory of its ribs, its knees, its shoulder-blades, offered it a series of rooms in which it had one time or another slept, while the unseen walls, shifting and adapting themselves to the shape of each successive room that I remembered, whirled around in the dark. [...] [M]y body, the side upon which I was laying, faithful guardians of a past which my mind should never have forgotten, brough back before my eyes that glimmering flame of the night-light in its urn-shaped bowl of Bohemian glass that hung by chains from the ceiling, and the chimney-piece of Siena marble in my bedroom at Combray, in my grandparents' house, in those far distant days which at this moment I imagined to be in the present without being able to picture them exactly. (Proust, 1992, pp. 5–6)

Bergson distinguished between recollection memory (*souvenir-image*) and habitual memory (*mémoire-habitude*). The latter does not represent the past but rather re-enacts it unconsciously in a bodily practical implementations. The past is implicitly contained in the present sensory impression and may unfold out of the body memory to form a conscious remembering (cf. Fuchs, 2021, pp. 222–223). Autobiographical memory hides a deeper un-vanishing layer of bodily experience. The same is unfortunately true for negative and traumatic experiences, for example, in the form of flashbacks. Spontaneous memory (*mémoire involontaire*) is, similarly to a dream, an intense, real-like recollection that appears briefly to disappear just moments later. It is not an image. The

source of intensity lies in the sensory experience. An Israeli writer, Nava Semel, describes the phenomenon as follows: "Suddenly, a smell of roasted chestnuts pierced his entire body. For a split second, he remembered walking down the street, holding his mother's hand. She was patiently peeling chestnuts, her hands full of soot. This must have been before the war" (Semel, 2001, p. 19). The memory disappears almost immediately, and it cannot be recalled, but the narrator of the story has already lost his appetite for chestnuts. He has only one sentence left of his mother: "Your brothers," she replied when he had asked who was on the photograph. "Where had they disappeared to?" he used to wonder as a child. Even if knowledge is full of secrets, writes Semel, it still exists in every pore and every cell of our bodies.

Literature as Inspiration and Model for Dream-Talk in Psychoanalysis

Dream-talk draws inspiration from poetic language, which links the sensual with the figurative and goes beyond semantic limitations. Freud passionately read great literature. For many analysts, such as Bion, Winnicott, Ogden, Loewald, and Parsons, literature is more than inspiration. It is a tool employed in clinical work. Literature is an instrument that enables the interpenetration of reality and fantasy, which, in turn, helps the analytic couple find adequate words. It creates and maintains a transitory space that gives us strength to live. The above-mentioned psychoanalysts don't utilize literature to decipher symbolic meanings with psychoanalytic concepts. Instead, they used it to find the right tone for improvisations and to draw closer to this particular experience, well-known from everyday analytic practice, yet so hard to put into words. It enables us to come nearer to the experience of uttering the hum of language and listening to it. Describing nuances, hues, and cracks is challenging; making them audible and visible is even harder.

The selfless quality of literature and the transitional purposelessness of an analytic session allow readers and analysands, respectively, to re-play their lives. Speaking is not just about reporting or narrating; the act of speaking is involved in unconscious staging. Facial expressions and gestures play an important role in the process. When patients talk about themselves, the act of speaking enables them to relive the narrated events and enhance them with fantasies. As a result, the past events gain vibrancy and intensity. According to Winnicott, transitory space, where fantasies mixed with reality are developed, has the capacity to transform existence into a creative life and should not be fully abandoned. Loewald writes about the dialectic of fantasy and reality, which are not set in opposition. These are, of course, not fantasies that should be given up, but fantasies that are indeed necessary in the development of object love (cf. Loewald, 1975, p. 298). Winnicott contrasts pure factual life or compulsive fantasizing with the third, transitory realm of both dreaming and trying.

There are patients who are unable to dream due to an acute trauma or deprivation, psychosomatic illness, state of nothingness, autistic spectrum, and severe perversion or addiction (Ogden, 2007, p. 576). In such cases, we don't pursue genealogical understanding through uncovering, but rather contain our patients in an aethreral, delicate way to allow them to accept traumatic experiences.

It is not a coincidence that Ogden, who conceptualized the autistic-contiguous position, was deeply concerned with poetry. On the one hand, sound and rhythm have a containing function, on the other, they reach much deeper than semantics. They move us. In his clinical practice, Ogden focused less on content and more on talking as a process, the effects of language, and the ways in which people use language to express themselves. What I am looking for is a poetic moment that may take on a number of different shapes. Here is an example: A colleague of mine repeated to his patient, who was unable to break away from her busy, hectic lifestyle, the following sentence from her story: "I once took my granddaughter in a stroller for a walk to an area I had never been to before." By emphasizing an "unknown area," the analyst allowed the patient to feel that she had dared to enter her early childhood "area" using experience with her granddaughter, which had so far been emotionally inaccessible to her. The fact that the poetic moment was directly linked with a sensory experience, mediated by the sound of the analyst's voice, led to the condensation of language and gave it a glow.

When my patient, Svenja, fully occupied me with her to-do lists, I remembered an Emily Dickinson poem that resembles a list but is significantly different:

To make a prairie it takes a clover and one bee,
One clover, and a bee.
And revery.
The revery alone will do,
If bees are few. (Dickinson, 1960, p. 710)

When I recited these verses to my patient, she interrupted me: "I can't do that. I don't have reveries and I don't dream, but yesterday I took a nap in the afternoon and dreamt of my childhood friend, Pia. She is no longer around. I woke up with a very sore neck." My patient was astonished at what "came out of her." We then had an unprecedented talk about pain and sadness.

I remember another patient who exuded austerity and lifelessness with her entire body. She lost her mother early on. Once, when she got sick, we talked over the phone for an entire week. After her usual dose of complaints, she started telling me about her grandfather from her childhood: "He has always been and still is so full of light despite being ninety." Her transformed voice made me beam inside. I then remembered my favorite poem by Osip Mandelstam:

This is what I most want
un-pursued, alone
to reach beyond the light
that I am furthest from.
And for you to shine there-
no other happiness-
and learn, from starlight,
what its fire might suggest.
A star burns as a star,
light becomes light,
because our murmuring
strengthens us, and warms the night.
And I want to say to you
my little one, whispering,
I can only lift you towards the light
by means of this babbling. (Mandelstam, 2000)

I simply said: "You were also so full of light, talking about your grandfather, and you moved me deeply." P: "And I felt as if you were sitting by my bed for an entire week and listened to me, until I was well again."

Drawing on Ogden, I understand the state of reverie as well as dream-talk with patients as an experience of becoming alive, when emotional experiences can be dreamt and articulated. I am referring to supporting patients in their ability to dream of their own experiences.

The pathological aspect of the autistic-contiguous position consists in the withdrawal, fragmentation, or "encapsulation" of unbearable states that have a bodily dimension. It is important to reveal this side of the patient and to follow it in therapy. To work with the patient to find adequate words/forms/images for it, but to let them remain unsaturated. We all have an inner secret space of solitude, never fully engaged in communication, always unnamed or not named directly, which should nonetheless be acknowledged in therapy. It is an attempt to approach our traumatized, autistic, and neglected patients. It is, however, equally important to search for and identify this type of access with all of our patients. Most of them and most of us are familiar with emotional states, which were covered up during our lives and couldn't articulate themselves, and as a result became unavailable as a source of vitality.

It wasn't until the 1960s that a number of analysts, such as Tustin, Ogden, Anzieu, and Kristeva, drew attention to the sensory components of an experience and discovered in them the source of nondiscursive, poetic use of language (cf. Rothbarth, 2021, p. 231). The words as "tonal voices" are mainly resonance, echo, consonances and dissonances, and reverberations. "[T]he infinity of sound reverberations and puns [...] form[s] the texture of the unconscious" (Dolar, 2006, pp. 161, 158).

In her work with autistic children, Frances Tustin discovered that they don't know how to play and they don't have elaborate fantasies. As a result, it is difficult for them to talk about their sensory, pleasurable, or terrifying experiences, and to display them. Poetry is particularly well-suited for expressing such experiences. Tustin called psychoanalysis "a kind of poetic science." She believed that everyone who works with autistic children should have access to the poetic experience (Tustin, 1986, p. 20).

My German patient, Marie, was always happy to hear me recite a fragment of a Polish poem. She would repeat the lines rhythmically while swinging her arms and legs. It was as if in these moments, her motionless body underwent rhythmization. Not one she asked about the meaning of the lines.

Let us now return to my initial clinical question: How do bodily experiences, which are at the same time subjective and referring to the outside world, emerge from the biological body? This question is particularly relevant in the case of patients with autistic tendencies, as they particularly suffer from distorted, unstable, and inconsistent body perception. In the process of dream-talking, images and sounds are used to build a bridge between body and mind, a between a sensory impression, experiencing it, and relations with others. This way, primary expressions are created. The basic substrate of images that present (and not represent) are not linguistic conventions, but rather bodily, motoric, and sensory experiences condensed in a body image perceived as "a prototype of internal images" (Fellmann, 1991, p. 62). Articulation precedes representation. Situated midway between finding and inventing, it opens up the reality by transforming the experienced life into expressive forms. This concept, aligned with Winnicott's thought, was formulated by a hermeneutic philosopher, Ferdinand Fellmann, who developed the notion of symbolic pragmatism. Reaching beyond communication patterns, he studied the structures of primary formations of expressions. He believed that situational and occasional meanings are expressed in language "predominantly in evocative or poetic speech" (Fellmann, 1991, p. 14). The figurative quality of poetic language predates linguistic discursiveness because of its unmediated presence and multiplicity of references. This is the primary shaping of the lived experience that allows people to first distance themselves from the excesses of affects and impulses.

Reverie is not a thought in a cognitive sense, but rather a creative moment, during which density occurs, similarly to poetry. It may or may not happen. If a creative moment occurs, it may be powerful enough to encourage the patient to leave the entanglement in their own patterns. Dream-talk is a psychoanalytic equivalent to maternal reverie. It gives fluidity to unshakable beliefs and ready-made language. They become unconscious, which, in turn, restores richness, vibrance, and depth to emotional experiences. Talking-as-dreaming searches, stumbles, and stutters, yet it is capable of getting right to the heart of the matter. It speaks through the gaps and addresses what has not been articulated. The power of an expressive occurrence stems from its anchoring in bodily experiences. On the other hand, words articulate and open up states that have not yet been represented, by outlining and naming them. To use Merleau-Ponty's notion, it is the miracle of creative expression, which allows a still-silent experience to self-express.

It is worth distinguishing between listening and hearing. In listening, we look for meaning; in hearing, we look for something that announces itself in the voice, going beyond meaning. Hearing is openness to something uncertain, fleeting, and attached to the voice. Michael Parsons introduced the distinction between hearing and abstracting the meaning. He was inspired by the poet Seamus Heaney, who believed that in poems should not be explored for meanings, but rather became an echo chamber for the sound of the poem (cf. Parsons, 2007, p. 1446). It is a mimetic way of hearing with the whole body. "[W]hen we hear inside us the poem which is the rain-stick, we become the rain-stick" (Parsons, 2007, p. 1447). Parsons asks, how can analysts apply this type of hearing to patients. It involves hearing through the poem's rhythm to the patient's approach to life and reality at the given moment. The analyst's dynamic alertness allows them to bridge the gap between feelings and interpretations. This is not countertransference, but rather a readiness for being deeply touched by the analysis in a way that expands our psychic capacities. For example, when Parsons's patient realizes that he has had twenty-five years of an unproductive life, the analyst has to rediscover in himself the ability to accept and face losses (and not just contemplate them). A particular analysis encourages the analyst to engage in personal psychic work on their own circumstances, which, in turn, allows him to better comprehend the pain and loss experienced by their patient. According to Parsons:

> The intimations of mortality are my own, and facing them is personal work in an area beyond countertransference. But this personal psychic work fold back into the internal setting that exists in my mind for this analysis. This gives [my patient] Mr W's life a depth and texture for me that lets me hear more in what he says, and helps me know more about his pain. (Parsons, 2007, p. 1454)

I remember a patient who was friendly, bright, and intelligent. At the same time, I gradually started to sense that there was something elusive about him, something I was unable to name, hidden in his movements and gestures … When I paid more attention to my own voice, to how I addressed him, I discovered that I had been adding a hint of gentle irony to everything I said. I described the situation to my patient, but refrained from offering interpretations or drawing conclusions. After a few seconds of dead silence, I heard: "It's because I feel so weak and stupid."

Functions of Dream-Talk

In the following segment of my chapter, I will briefly describe the functions of dream-talk in the analytic process. They include: 1) Natality 2) play and eternity of the moment, 3) self-agency and the creative work of an analytic couple, and 4) transgression.

Natality

In analysis, we are used to devoting a lot of time to limitation, renunciation, finiteness, and regret. As Heidegger puts it, to be-in-the-world, we have to accept the being-toward-death. However, an equally essential component is the natality of a human being as the source of the new, the promise, and the future. It is an opportunity to see the world with new eyes. To be born means to emerge from the world and for the world. The world is already formed but it will never be fully formed. It consumes us at first, but then it opens us to the universe of possibilities (cf. Merleau-Ponty, 1973, p. 89).

To be accepted without the possessive gesture, the New needs a "Midwife of Becoming," or Plato's *khôra.* He understands it as a conceptless matrix, a pulsation giving the world its contours, shapes, and boundaries. Plato's *khôra* is a kind of a container without any properties. Its all-receptivity resembles Bion's reverie mother as well as Winnicott's mother who is capable of adequately responding to her infant precisely because she agrees to being used. In a creative process of coming into being, she makes her breast available to her baby the moment it is capable of discovering it. Mother-Khôra is capable of waiting for the right moment. This way, time is introduced. Anxiety and other difficult feelings should be experienced and kept, in accordance with Bion's negative capability. As a result, a continuity of existence is created, which evokes the sense of being alive. Mother-Khôra's receptiveness does not distinguish between passivity and activity. Following Bion, positions of activity and passivity alternate. Similarly, Winnicott's formlessness contains both elements: creative potential of the experience and traumatic threat of disintegration. A defensive reflex of the latter results in a fixation of the form and a blocking out of the creative potential. Such patients fantasize but they don't dream.

Dream-talk is characterized by a passive–active receptivity that allows the other, a patient, to touch us and get under our skin. This form of communication enables the other to deposit something inside of us, with an unconscious hope that we will carry it with us for a while, transform it, and return it reshaped. This is the positive component of projective identification, or, as Derrida calls it, hospitality. It entails openness to accept the other devoid of the possessive gesture. Only this experience gives an analyst the right to analyze.

Play and Eternity of the Moment

In my work with adult patients, I always search for a possibility to play and create together. This level corresponds with play in child analysis. It is frequently referred to but rarely practiced in adult analysis. It requires sensitive listening and creativity in the talking cure.

A patient of mine has recently told me about her dream. She was lying between spaghetti and tomato sauce on a shelf in a supermarket, while I spoke to her by way of a loudspeaker. She ended up not buying anything but the cashier made her pay anyway. Outraged, she wrote a letter to Melanie Klein who responded with a demand to be left alone since she is already dead. Of course, I had a lot of ideas for interpretation, but my initial thought was that this dream was like a work of art. I was happy to hear that my patient dreams in this way, similarly to a mother happy to see what her child had built out of blocks. My interpretation was: "What a great dream!"

Dream-talk involves silence, stuttering, and mumbling, sometimes of decisive importance. If we treat this level seriously, we will see that the "classic" interpretation of defense and conflict does not reach it or omits it. Reverie manifests itself in many ways: with words, gestures, images, sounds, or gazes. Why do I prefer to discuss dream-talk, rather than the earlier-discussed interpretation offered from the position of reverie? To allow time and maintain the openness for longer. Dream-talk is stretchy; it opens up the time between being moved by something and responding to it – the time for developing fantasies.

Proust describes a timeless, present experience of enjoying the moment capable of reconciling being-toward-death with a traumatic past:

> This explains why it was that my anxiety on the subject of my death had ceased at the moment when I had unconsciously recognized the taste of the little madeleine, since the being which at the moment I had been an extra-temporal being. [...] [T]he miracle of an analogy [...] had the power to perform that task which had always defeated the efforts of my memory and my intellect, the power to made me rediscover days that were long past, the Time that was Lost. (Proust, 2003, pp. 262–263)

Proust discovered eternity in art. In psychoanalytic dream-talk, we sometimes experience these eternities of the moment.

Sense of Self-Agency and the Creative Work of a Psychoanalytic Couple

According to Ogden, during a session, analyst and patient try to speak in a way that conveys a sense of the patient being alive at that moment, to the extent of the latter's capabilities. "[T]he analyst must be attuned to what the patient is doing with language, as well as all that he is unable to do. Language is not simply a medium for the expression of the self; it is integral to the creation of the self" (B.H. Ogden & T.H. Ogden, 2013, p. 9). Benjamin Ogden and Thomas Ogden focus on the use of language and its impact on the analytic couple in a specific moment, rather than on hidden meanings. Thomas Ogden makes a generalization by moving on to the question of analytic work with particular patients. Voice expresses the condition of being human under particular circumstances (cf. Ogden, 2007, p. 586).

Dream-talk often allows patient to discover her or his bodily self. In the course of an interaction during a successful session, patient and analyst – each in their own way and on their own level – become artists and mediums for one another. Beneficial sessions/phases allow them to co-create a fantasy life that, in turn, shapes the patient's conduct in his actual life (cf. Loewald, 1975, p. 297). This fantasy creation, in which both the patient and the analyst participate, has been described in a number of ways. Bion imagined a shared weaving of thoughts without a thinker, Winnicott invented the "squiggle game," Ogden – the analytic third. It is a happening consisting of an interpenetration of passive receptions and active answers. Hartmut Rosa introduced the notion of "medio-passivity" (Rosa, 2020, p. 29). It is a state that emerges

> when, for example, people dance, perform or play music or theater together [...]. When it becomes impossible to distinguish between those who conduct and those who receive; they are simultaneously both. One is so absorbed by the event that being affected by something else and responding to it become one half-active-passive act. Resonance as an intense entry into a relationship cannot be forced. Patience and exercise are needed on the one hand, and reverie, freedom, serenity on the other. (Rosa, 2020, p. 30)

Merleau-Ponty also indicates a form of a successful fusion in speaking and listening:

> When I am listening, it is not necessary that I have an auditory perception of the articulated sounds but that the conversation pronounces itself within me. It summons me and grips me; it envelops and inhabits me to the point that I cannot tell what comes from me and what from it. Whether speaking or listening, I project myself into the other person, I introduce him into my own self. (Merleau-Ponty, 1973, p. 19)

When we leave the "ready-made language" during an analytic session, boundaries between the speaker and the listener become fluid. The resulting intersection is a surprising, and perhaps disturbing and confusing encounter of two individuals leading to a mutual transformation. It is the effect of the collective work of the analytic couple.

Transgression

Transgression is not just the question of working through one's relationships with parents, but rather, following Kierkegaard, a "recalling ahead," a creative process that calls something new into being. Transgression of what is actually given includes the experience of trembling and the negative capability, "that is, when a man is capable of being in uncertainties, mysteries, doubts, without any irritable reaching after fact and reason" (Keats, qt. in Bion, 1995, p. 125). Post-scientific psychoanalysis, represented by Lacan, Laplanche, Bion, Winnicott, Ogden, and others, does not renunciate metaphysical desire or the experience of transcending what is given. Not everything can be explained without stripping life of its mystery and unpredictability. Winnicott and Bion both acknowledged the limits of enlightenment. A psychoanalytic situation may be seen as a transitory space where the visible intertwines with the invisible, the audible with the inaudible, the familiar with the uncanny, the intimate with the distant, the conscious with the unconscious, and the articulated with the unspeakable.

Case Study: Marie – from Biological Body to Bodily Self

I would like to conclude my chapter by taking a closer look at different aspects of corporeality from the viewpoint of the notion of dream-talk, using the example of my clinical work with the above-mentioned Marie, whose mother had suffered from a mental illness. Negligence, sexual violence, and mental abuse have left Marie severely traumatized. She didn't speak, and she couldn't feel her own body. She initiated a form of communication based on gestures and facial expressions, which led to a lengthy process of developing a bodily self. In fact, her dependence on this elementary communication clearly showed me how I had unintentionally attuned myself to her by using facial expressions and gestures that contributed to the processes of transference and countertransference.

With hindsight, I can now distinguish five cornerstone elements of this process. I will examine them in the following order: 1) calls, appeals, and their reception, linked with the bodily presence of the analyst; 2) description of the elementary states without directly addressing Marie, such as "you are ... ," or "you are feeling ... ," and definitely short of explanatory interpretations, "this is because ... "; 3) sharing experiences; 4) speech acts and their processing; and 5) dream-talk that supported the development of a new sense of self. In some aspects, my approach to working with Marie resembled the work of Ann Alvarez, which came to my attention only after I had formulated my concept.

Calls and Appeals

Marie would initiate a call, trying to energize me with gaze and "mm-hmm?" to make contact and draw my attention to her: "are you there?" If I hadn't responded immediately to her facial expressions and uttered sounds, her face became motionless and darkened. When she withdrew and grew lifeless, I did what she had done: "Hallo, are you there?" In her case and with other patients incapable of listening or feeling, a simple invitation to establish contact has worked in an invigorating way.

Description of Elementary Experiences without an Addresser

I started by describing elementary sensory experiences "into space," without addressing Marie directly. I was careful to depart from meanings as well as feelings. If I said, for example: "you look sad," Marie would immediately react with: "How do you know?" and withdraw into herself. Even a simple comment "you are crying" was too much for her. When I said: "A large tear is coursing down your cheek," she wiped it, saying: "It's not there anymore," and started talking. I tried to touch just the very surface of senses, without going any further and deeper.

Marie would join me when I spoke into space. For example: "Street noise is very loud today" was her own observation, not a direct derivation from mine: "It is colder here today than yesterday." She liked it because it allowed for a larger distance between us while carefully building a connection. It was a form of speaking without a clear authorship. When we talked, I rarely said "you," because she would immediately regard it as a reproach and back away. For a long time, she was incapable of feeling sad or saying it, but she was able to describe her state as "gray and tight." It took her three years to say: "I think I am starting to understand what you mean when you ask me 'how does it feel'."

Sharing Experiences

The next step was about sharing experiences. I was revealing my own thoughts and sensations to my patient from time to time, inviting her into my thinking, feeling, and speaking processes. In a more advanced stage of the analysis, Marie worked up the courage to ask me about my own feelings. For example, whether I ever cried at the doctor's office or was unable to fall asleep. She would find a slightly delayed, affirmative answer satisfactory (if I actually had experienced this). It would visibly affect her and make her feel more alive. She realized that others had comparable experiences to her own. It was like being invited to participate in a shared universe. A sense of belonging to a greater whole has a therapeutic effect that Winnicott was aware of.

Marie started to discover her difficult experiences in me, someone capable of both experiencing and referring to the experiences. From a clinical perspective, it is important to hold off with returning patients' projections (cf. Alvarez & Furgiuele, 1997, pp. 123–139) and to continuously re-regulate the delicate balance between openness, intensity, and distance instead. If my facial expression suggested distance, Marie took it as ultimate abandonment. She was able to tell me later: "When you distance yourself, I put in a lot of effort to provoke you. My mother wouldn't react to anything, so I provoked her to know where she was." Competence, or internalized setting as I called it elsewhere (Kobylinska-Dehe, 2019, p. 532), helped me find the right balance at most times.

On Speech Acts and Bodily Processing

We know that psychoanalysis, French psychoanalysis in particular, was greatly influenced by structural linguistics. Contrary to structuralists, phenomenologists did not study linguistic structures, but rather the "expressive speech" anchored in gestures, perception, and the spontaneous body. It is easy for psychoanalysts to follow these phenomenological ideas.

Bodily talking and processing our relationship in the "here and now" helped me make progress with Marie. "How" we talked was more important than "what" we said: too much, too fast, too quietly, "I need a moment to think … something has touched me." Descriptions of what was happening, such as "we are just starting to get entangled," brought relaxation. For a while we stayed at the level of process interpretation, as Reinhard Plassmann called it. When I asked her during a much later session: "What do you think is happening here?" Marie replied: "I am messing with your head and confusing you, just like my father did with me. And you are like a helpless child, you don't stand a chance." There was no need for me to add anything.

Dream-Talk and the Basic Melody of the Soul

Marie started to live in her own body. She was no longer overwhelmed by an excess of stimuli and was sometimes able to create images representing her states during sessions. In the later period, when she was already laying on the couch, she was able to relax a little and speak from that position: "I lived my life in a constriction and wasn't aware of it. But if you are contracted you cannot swim." An image emerged from a bodily experience. Marie connected sensory perception with word image in a fascinating way. She also produced free associations when one of us did something that resembled "interpretation as reverie." It is a combination of sensory perception, a not-fully defined image, and a welcoming into the world. What emerges is a figure that is simultaneously: fleeting and leaving a mark, like a dream.

Toward the end of his life, Winnicott put forth an idea that the ability to be alone and the sense of being real both require the support of an unknown and invisible environment. This is what I have in mind by the notion of being welcomed into the world.

One time, Marie came into the office and said: "It got brighter It is now lighter." Indeed, it started to clear up outside. Marie repeated a modified version of the sentence: "Things got brighter in my life. I didn't realize it was so dark in my life. My sense of smell has somehow changed too. I am starting to smell the seasons." She wasn't able to put it into words before because she didn't feel that something was missing or that things could be different. She still has problems but it ceased to be so gray, heavy, and sad. The turning point was the emergence of a new feeling, a basic melody of the soul, and the budding capacity for reverie that came with it. But before she could experience this feeling and express it, she had to feel it with her body.

Of course, I had tried different interpretations before discovering the elementary level of calls and descriptions. At the level of interpretation, I was unable to reach my patient at all. She had felt persecuted and reacted with extreme agitation and resistance. An interpretation had been impossible until we started building together an embodied mental space and laying foundations for a human capacity for relationships (Alvarez).

Conclusion: Environment as a sensory Surroundings and Space of Acceptance

My final clinical example will illustrate the importance of the sensory environment in connection to the analyst's receptivity in the process of transformation and highlight once more the role of dream-talk. According to Winnicott, a responsive and holding environment activates self-healing powers.

I often kept a vase full of flowers on the floor of my office. My patients could see them from the couch, out of the corner of an eye. I would gaze at the flowers in a moment of reverie. They reminded me of the changing seasons, and provided comfort and calm during the most challenging sessions. I believe that they did the same for some of my patients.

Anna was deeply confused about her sexual identity; she presented herself as a shapeless lump, lifeless, and mute. She would sometimes fall into states that brought to mind a terrified infant. Following one of our sessions, I found a note on the couch entitled "Secrets." I managed to decipher these scribbled words:

The flowers were there from the very beginning.
Different ones every time. Single flowers raised their heads
above the large vase. Or, in small groups,
performed their own colorful dances
and seemed to be smiling.
She didn't know how to call them.
Initially, she seemed to barely notice them. Flowers were simply a part of the great Outside
She once lost.
The shape of it, behind the dark drapes,

she vaguely imagined
Her gaze focused only on what
had promised to hold her.
Then, when the fog had lifted, she was at a loss of words,
To say something.
And when one day, for the first time
she gazed into the eye of the flower, something
had opened up in her abdomen and colors
reached her, she fell silent.
She even turned her head away, ashamed.
And since then, she gazed stealthily
at the procession of bouquets, narrowing her eyes
And trying to touch their dance, as she passed by
discretely, her actions unnoticed.
As the sunny days grew long enough to
remember the surroundings in the daylight,
and she learned to not lose track of things even in the fog.
She let her gaze rest
on the flowers longer
She even tilted her head a little
when she sat down.
She noticed in passing that this movement has almost gotten lost
When she got up
that it might have helped her run up to simultaneously
put both legs on the couch,
which color she had forgotten
the moment she left the room.
She noticed it and smiled.

My patient describes the process of sensory perception in unique poetic words as gazing, touching, moving, opening of abdomen, disappearance off a heavy drape, and an acquired ability to not get lost even in her own darkness. At the end, there is a restrained courage to present herself and an amusing moment when Anna notices her own subversiveness.

It would be difficult to find a better conclusion ending than Anna's description that illustrates the process of subjectivizing bodily experiences using dream-talk on the psychoanalyst's couch.

References

Alvarez, A. & Furgiuele, P. (1997): Speculations on Components in the Infant's Sense of Agency: The Sense of Abundance and the Capacity to Think in Parentheses. In: Reid, S. (Ed.): *Developments in Infant Observation: The Tavistock Model*. London: Routledge.

Bion, W. R. (1995): *Attention and Interpretation*. Lanham, MD: Rowman & Littlefield Publishers.

Dickinson, E. (1960): *The Complete Poems of Emily Dickinson*. Ed. by T. H. Johnson. Boston/Toronto: Little, Brown & Company.

Dolar, M. (2006): *A Voice and Nothing More*. Boston: Massachusetts Institute of Technology.

Fellmann, F. (1991): *Symbolischer Pragmatismus. Hermeneutik nach Dilthey*. Reinbek: Rowohlt.

Freud, S. (1905d): Three Essays on the Theory of Sexuality. SE VII, 123–246.

Freud, S. (1914c): The Moses of Michelangelo. SE XIII, 122–150.

Frost, R. (1942): *A Witness Tree*. New York: Henry Holt.

Fuchs, T. (2021): *In Defense of the Human Being: Foundational Questions of an Embodied Anthropology*. Oxford: Oxford University Press.

Goldschmidt, G. (2006): *Als Freud das Meer sah. Freud und die deutsche Sprache*. Trans. by B. Grosse. Zurich: Ammann.

Kobylinska-Dehe, E. (2019): Vom Leib zum phantasmatischen Körper-Bewegung, Berührung, Phantasie. *Psyche – Z Psychoanal*, 73, 523–545.

Kobylinska-Dehe, E. (2021): Gegen die Ausdünnung der Erfahrung. Psychoanalyse und die responsive Phänomenologie. In: Schellhammer, B. (Ed.): *Zwischen Phänomenologie und Psychoanalyse*. München: Nomos.

Loewald, H. W. (1971): On Motivation and Instinct Theory. *Psychoanalytic Study of the Child*, 26, 91–128.

Loewald, H. W. (1975): Psychoanalysis as an Art and the Fantasy Character of the Psychoanalytic Situation. *JAPA*, 23(2), 277–299.

Lombardi, R. (2016): *Formless Infinity: Clinical Explorations of Matte Blanco and Bion*. London/New York: Routledge.

Mandelstam, O. (2000): This is What I Most Want. Trans. by A. S. Kline. www.poetryintranslation.com.

Merleau-Ponty, M. (1973): *The Prose of the World*. Trans. by J. O'Neill. Evanston: Northwestern University Press.

Merleau-Ponty, M. (2012): *Phenomenology of Perception*. Trans. by D. A. Landes. New York: Routledge.

Ogden, B. H. & Ogden, T. H. (2013): *The Analyst's Ear and the Critic's Eye. Rethinking Psychoanalysis and Literature*. New York: Routledge.

Ogden, T. H. (2007): On Talking-as-Dreaming. *Int J Psychoanal*, 88(3), 575–589.

Parsons, M. (2007): Raiding the Inarticulate: The Internal Analytic Setting and Listening Beyond Countertransference. *Int J Psychoanal*, 88, 1441–1456.

Proust, M. (1992): *In Search of Lost Time, Vol. I: Swann's Way*. Trans. by C. K. S. Moncrieff, T. Kilmartin. New York: Random House Publishing Group.

Proust, M. (2003): *In Search of Lost Time, Vol. VI: Time Regained*. Trans. by A. Mayor, T. Kilmartin. New York: Random House Publishing Group.

Rosa, H. (2020): *Inne halten: Chronik einer Krise: Jenaer Corona-Gespräche*. Berlin: Theater der Zeit.

Rothbarth, S. (2021): Lyrik und autistisch-berührende Position. *Psyche – Z Psychoanal*, 75(3), 230–263.

Storck, T. & Brauner, F. (2021): *Körpergefühl*. Gießen: Psychosozial-Verlag.

Tokarczuk, O. (2018): Nobel Lecture: "The Tender Narrator". Trans. by J. Croft, A. Lloyd-Jones. Https://www.nobelprize.org/prizes/literature/2018/tokarczuk/lecture/.

Tustin, F. (1986): *Autistic Barriers in Neurotic Patients*. London: Karnac Books.

Chapter 10

The Via Regia of the Rhizome

Paths in the Unconscious of the Psychosomatic Body

Lutz Goetzmann

Royal Roads and Rhizomes

According to Freud, the interpretation of dreams represents the "the royal road to a knowledge of the unconscious activities of the mind" (cf. Freud, 1900, p. 608). Body experience could also be a "royal road" to the unconscious. In any case, the metaphor is often used in body therapy and embodiment literature (e.g., Rau-Luberichs, 2016, p. 213). Freud was probably referring to the Torah (Hamburger, 2013, p. 123), the book of Numbers 21:21–22 (the 4th book of Moses), which is called Bamidbar – in Hebrew "In the Desert":

> And Israel sent messengers unto Sihon, King of the Amorites, saying, Let me pass through thy land: we will not turn into the fields, or into the vineyards; we will not drink of the waters of the well: but we will go along by the king's highway, until we be past thy borders. (KJV)

Nevertheless, as reported in the book of Numbers, warfare ensued, and the land of the Amorite king was conquered. Another story about the royal road is that of the Egyptian king Ptolomaios I, formerly a general of Alexander the Great, who, according to Proclos (412–485 AD), is said to have asked Euclid of Alexandria (360–290 BC), when the latter's son was struggling with mathematics, if his teacher knew of no shorter, easier way than that of laboriously plowing through Euclid's own work Στοιχεῖα ("Elements"). Euclid had compiled and systematized the knowledge of arithmetic and geometry of his time. He thus depicted the structure of an exact science: statements and proofs derived from a stock of definitions, axioms, and postulates (e.g., that a distance can be drawn from one point to another). Up to modern times, this work was one of the most famous in world literature, but it apparently overwhelmed the prince and general's son.

Euclid is said to have answered the worried father negatively: There is no royal road to geometry ("μὴ εἶναι βασιλικὴν ἀτραπὸν ἐπί γεωμετρίαν") – no short, direct, and convenient way to understanding the matter. A royal road, by

DOI: 10.4324/9781003370130-10

the way, had also been built by Darius I between Anatolia and Persia to enable rapid communication and troop movement in the form of a royal "shortcut" (https://en.wikiquote.org/wiki/Euclid). Perhaps, however, Freud did not have a literal road in mind at all but rather thought of the proverbial phrase that goes back to a certain genre of books: "Via regia," according to Hamburger (2013, p. 123), was the name given to textbooks (or political instruction manuals) modeled on the first Carolingian Mirror of Princes. Emerald of Saint-Mihiel, the author, interpreted the aforementioned passage in Numbers 21:22 to mean that the via regia Moses intended to use to lead his people through the Land of Edom, namely, "the direct path of the elect to the heavenly fatherland, overcoming all obstacles." In this sense, the via regia is not a specific path but rather serves as a guide toward the desired goal: "The interpretation of dreams as via regia, that is, as a textbook" (Hamburger, 2013, p. 123). Deleuze and Guattari (cf. Kluge & Vogl, 2009, p. 308) speak of "royal science," meaning knowledge that is clearly ordered, solidly based, well-structured, for instance, by stable paths or routes, lines that lead directly from one point to the next, without deviations or the tendency to roam or wander. In their own cartography of knowledge, Deleuze and Guattari (1987 [1976]) use the image of the "rhizome": an underground passageway or tuber-like construction, a "labyrinth without a beginning and an end" (Kluge & Vogl, 2009, p. 308). These routes in a rhizome form the opposite of the royal road structure:

> First, a rhizome is a labyrinth, an underground passageway with few elements to distinguish it from the occidental story of the labyrinth. It is a labyrinth without a beginning and an end. If it is a labyrinth without a beginning and an end, it is also a labyrinth without Ariadne's thread, that is, without a center and a periphery. And, furthermore, a third character-istic is quite decisive for a rhizome: It is a ganged structure whose metrics – whose metrical order – is so perplexing that it is unclear how one can get from one element or position in the labyrinth to another. It is a system of shortcuts, of detours, and knows neither the straight, direct, nor correct path. These three elements: without a beginning and an end; without Ariadne's thread, that is, without a center and a periphery; and, finally, a system of corridors consisting only of shortcuts and detours, characterize a rhizome, which is, therefore, the place for the unforeseen encounter. (Kluge & Vogl, 2009, p. 313; here, the explanations of Joseph Vogl)

The paths to the unconscious are certainly more intricate, more "rhizo-matic," than a royal shortcut, a structured textbook, or a thoughtful model could ever hope for. These pathways traverse not only the territory of the dream, but also that of the body. The following essay is intended as a cartographic unfolding; it consists of two sections: In the first section, I present a psychoanalytic view of the relationship between body and soul/mind; I follow here the "royal science" of an abstract model that compiles and systematizes different psychoanalytic perspectives in the form of theoretical knowledge. In the second section, I report on applying this knowledge, but in the form of a nomadic travelogue, i.e., how to work with symptomatic bodily experiences in psychoanalytic therapy. Thus, I seek to combine the "royal science" of model and theory with the "nomadic science" of the rhizome, an endeavor whose dialectic provides insight into the unique, singular unconscious.

The General Model of Mental Functioning

Our starting point is Laplanche's "Fundamental Anthropological Situation," which he describes in the context of his "General Seduction Theory" (Laplanche, 2004; Laplanche, 2011, pp. 99–114). The basic idea is that there is an "unilateral" interference; the Other communicates a message to the child that seems puzzling for two reasons: The Other is unaware of the ambiguity, which stems from their own (sexual) pre-conscious; and the child cannot properly interpret this ambiguity. The child has to "translate" this enigmatic adult message into their own language. This translation takes place in two steps: First, the message is "inscribed" (or carved) in the child's psyche and thus retained below the "thin layer of consciousness." The place of this inscription is the "enclosed unconscious" (*inconscient enclavé*). The content is not yet represented, or, in Lacan's terminology, it is "real" (2021 [1974–1975]). Topologically, an "enclave of the real unconscious" ensues as a depository for the messages of the Other (like a "nest," i.e., where the psychic contents of the Other are collected in the subject; cf. de M'Uzan, 1989). It is the lair for the milk, the gaze, the voice, or organs of the Other: the nipples, the eyes, and the mouth. They are nonrepresented "things." Hegel (2010 [1830], §400) spoke of "simple" or "natural sensations" that can be understood as the result of confrontation with the Other. In contrast to the body, i.e., to material nature, these (unconscious, simple, and real) sensations belong to the "ideational"[1]: They constitute the ideational, immaterial side of matter.

In the *Encyclopedia of the Philosophical Sciences*, Hegel says the following:

> The soul is immaterial not only in itself but also for the general immateriality of nature, its simple ideational life. (Hegel, 2010 [1830], §389)

Lacan complements the ideational with the registers of the imaginary (i.e., figurative ideas) and the symbolic (i.e., linguistically composed thoughts). Figure 10.1 illustrates this "wholeness," composed of matter (M) and the ideational, i.e., the Real, the Imaginary, and the Symbolic (R, I, S).

We can characterize these registers of the psychic as follows (see Evans, 1996; also Lacan, 2021 [1974–1975]):

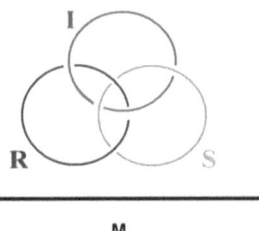

Figure 10.1 Matter (M)/ideality with the registers of the Real (R), Imaginary (I), and Symbolic (S).

1   The Real is something unspeakable; it cannot be imagined or represented; it lies beyond all appearances as the intangible of the unrepresented. It is the impossible, that which cannot be imagined or inserted into the symbolic order. This intractability is the traumatic moment of the Real. It is to be distinguished from reality (German *Wirklichkeit*) (Evans, 1996, p. 162).

2   The Imaginary is organized pictorially; it includes the world of phantasms, identifications, reflections, and body image. It lies between the Real, that is, the equally factual and intangible, nonrepresented reality of experience, and the symbolic in the sense of a linguistic order. The Imaginary develops in the subject's mirroring; the symbolic, which comes later, gives this dual reflection a linguistic meaning (Evans, 1996, p. 84 ff.)

3   The Symbolic is the order of language, discourse, structure, and laws (Evans, 1996, p. 203).

All bodily-material processes take place on the Matter (M) side: the excitations of the body, in particular, within the networks of the brain (here called "arousal"). The real sensations (R) and the pictorial and linguistic thoughts (S, I) take place on the ideational side, where the primordial translation performance also takes place: the translation of the real sensation into a pictorial idea (I) or a linguistically composed thought (S). The message, deposited in the enclave of the real unconscious, is like an "inner foreign body" that can be integrated only over time, i.e., by being translated into pictorial conceptions and linguistically composed thoughts. The translation achievements described by Laplanche basically consist not in translating the real (natural, simple) sensations into imaginary and symbolic ones (i.e., from one language into another), but in the translation variant(s) the subject chooses or appropriates. Interpretations are translation proposals at both levels, i.e., verbalizing real sensations (first level) or proposing translation variants in the imaginary–symbolic register (second level).

Thus, there are two types of translations in which afterwardness ("après-coup") is inscribed: The real sensation is translated (i.e., pictorially or linguistically determined) into the register of the imaginary and symbolic after the fact, possibly even only during adolescence or adulthood – or during analytic treatment, i.e., when the subject has acquired the corresponding mental maturity. In Hegel's dialectic, the real and simple sensation is indeed negated (like material excitement previously): On the one hand, it disappears; on the other hand, it is suspended, i.e., preserved, in pictorial conceptions and linguistically composed thoughts because of the "determinate negation." The second form of afterwardness consists of the choice of imaginary–symbolic translation variant (Laplanche, 1999, p. 260). For example, the sexual connotation of an enigmatic, seductive message the child receives from the Other may not be translated into sexualized semantics until adolescence (or even later). In this two-stage process, any translation represents a sort of mistranslation and, in this sense, a failed one.

Some aspects of the message, especially the traumatic ones, are untranslatable. They cannot be represented and elude the grasp of the symbolic. Especially in his later writings, Lacan (2016 [1962/1963], pp. 230) refers to such real remnants as "objects a," clearly only a placeholder for the unrepresentable. One can distinguish between "thing" and "object a": One can determine real sensations that refer to representable things (e.g., the partial objects mentioned above) imaginarily and symbolically. Thus, real sensations can be either representable things or nonrepresentable objects. Bion (1962, pp. 6) distinguishes between alpha and beta elements: Alpha elements are situated in a transformative intermediate stage and form the basis for pictorial ideas (I) and linguistically composed thoughts (S) (cf. Goetzmann, 2020). Beta elements (R) cannot be transformed but, according to Bion (1962, p. 23), accumulate on a "beta screen." So, alpha and beta sensations are real, whereby the former refer to representable things and the latter to nonrepresentable "objects a." In the enclave of the real unconscious, things are real, translatable, and representable alpha sensations; "objects a" are real, nontranslatable, and nonrepresentable beta sensations. However, the translation of the "thing" into the pictorial conception or the linguistically composed thought is probably never quite complete: Certain nonrepresentable remnants remain, which thus can likewise be called "objects a." A "thing" is never completely transformable, i.e., even an alpha perception (a "thing") contains a beta core (an "object a"): the never-emerging, "indivisible remainder" (Žižek, 2007). As mentioned, the beta "objects a" congregate in Bion's beta-screen, though they can also be "returned" to the Other in the form of a projective identification or discharged into the body as asymbolic symptoms. In this respect, the unconscious communication with the Other, who, among other things, serves as a container, is a thoroughly reciprocal one. The alpha thoughts formed in the preconscious can penetrate directly into consciousness – or they are repressed, for instance, at the behest of the superego. Thus, the ability to repress creates a (repressed) unconscious, which is not real but has an imaginary–symbolic nature. Its contents enter the subject's consciousness indirectly, in a veiled way, as dream images, slips of the tongue, symbolic bodily symptoms, or wrongdoings.

The question is: How do feelings fit into this translation landscape? One could conceive of feelings as prelinguistic, imageless thoughts that arise on a purely phenomenal, prepositional level (Demmerling, 2021). Even when a feeling is present, it is not yet pictorially or linguistically grasped or determined. Herrmann Schmitz (2020, p. 30), who founded the "New Phenomenology" movement, described feelings as "spatially discharged atmospheres." In this respect, one could distinguish between real sensations, on the one hand, and felt (phenomenal), imagined, and symbolic thoughts, on the other hand. As soon as a feeling becomes a dream image or a linguistic statement ("I am sad," "I am happy") in waking life, it loses its pure phenomenality and takes on an imaginary or symbolic quality. The phenomenal world of feelings thus emerges in the interface from the real (sensation) to the imaginary–symbolic (figurative and linguistic thoughts).

Laplanche (2004) illustrated his model using a diagram taken from Dejours' *Le corps d'abord* (2001) (see Figure 10.2): The mental apparatus consists of two parts (A and B). On the one hand, they are separate from each other; on the other hand, there is a porous transition zone that allows the translation of real sensations (in the enclave of the real unconscious, i.e., the enclosed unconscious, (B) and the preconscious or repressed unconscious (A). In the case of a mature, well-structured neurosis, Part A is much more extensive than Part B. In borderline cases or psychoses, Part B may even gain the upper hand. Figure 10.2 shows a general model of mental functioning according to Laplanche (2004) and Dejours (2001), respectively, with the integration of both the psychoanalytic (Laplanche, Lacan, Bion) and philosophical perspectives (Hegel).

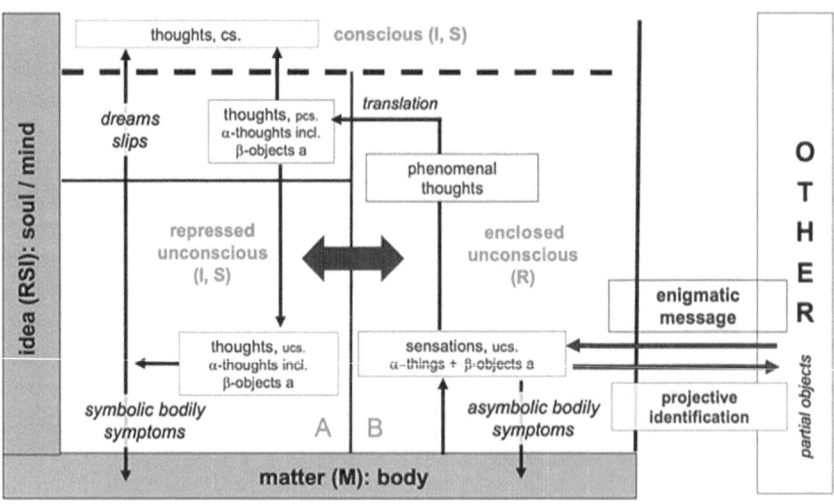

Figure 10.2 General model of mental functioning.

The Psychosomatic Totality

Against the background of this model, we developed the "axis of psycho-somatic totality" (Goetzmann et al., 2020), which includes the Borromean ensemble of ideality (R, S, I), i.e., the indeterminate and determinate sensations, and matter (M), i.e., the natural body. Thus, space also has different qualities, namely, material and Borromean. Outside the Borromean space (R, S, I) lies nature (body, M): The material space of the body is the outsideness of nature. In the body, material excitations take place, whose ideal aspects are the (initially real) sensations. The material excitations or the "sum of excitations" (*sommes d'excitations*; Sami-Ali, 2006, p. 6) are negated or canceled out in the ideational sensations. On the other hand, bodily excitations constitute the material aspect of sensations: They can spread throughout the body or in certain regions. That is where the sensations are canceled or negated. The whole ideational nature of soul and spirit is held together by the consistency of the imaginary. Thus, the "axis of psycho-somatic totality" rests, as it were, in an imaginary space, i.e., within the imaginary space of the Borromean body (or, as phenomenology would say: the "body" [*Leib*]; cf. Schmitz, 2011) various forms of psychosomatic symptom formation can be described and topologically assigned to an "axis."

One distinguishes between the symbolic and asymbolic poles of the axis: At the symbolic pole, body symbols are formed in the form of "hysterical" conversion symptoms; at the asymbolic pole I, the bodily symptoms are stripped of all symbolic meaning – they are asymbolic, operative, or mechanical. Figure 10.3 shows the "axis of psychosomatic totality."

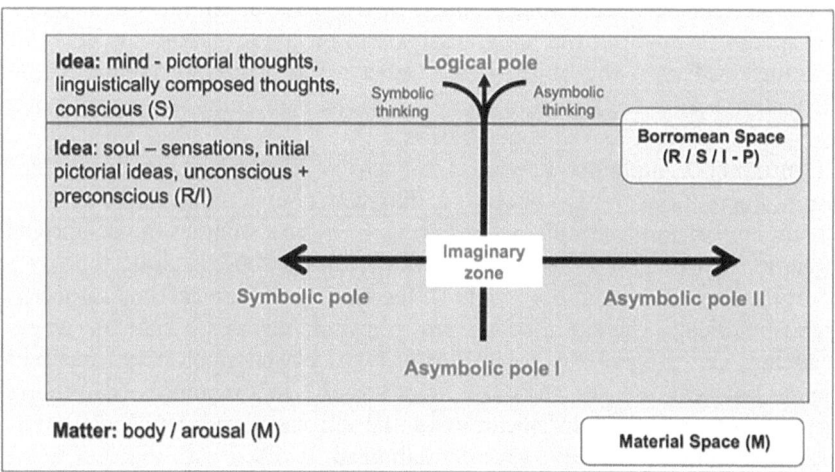

Figure 10.3 The axis of psychosomatic totality.

The symbolic pole is located in area A (cf. Figure 10.2), i.e., in the territory of the *repressed unconscious*. The latter can form both mental symptoms (e.g., in dreams, fantasies), behavioral symptoms (e.g., wrong actions, slips of the tongue, acting out), and physical symptoms (disturbances of bodily functions), which develop from the dialectic of the wish (need, demand, desire) and the difficulty of its realization (e.g., as a result of a prohibition). The bodily symptoms (or body symbols) are manifest, material symptoms (M) resulting from the latent modification of the imaginary body image, for instance, in the form of motor or sensory function failures in the interplay between wish and prohibition. On the side of the symbolic pole lies the mature defense style of repression: The subject can differentiate between themselves and the Other or between objects. Accordingly, the subject's experience is triadic, and their imaginary space remains largely intact. All symptoms, whether mental, behavioral, or physical, have an alpha character, i.e., they are symbolic–imaginary translations of the real, of things that are based as alpha sensations on the (enigmatic) messages of the Other.

The asymbolic pole I lies in the realm of the real, i.e., of the *enclosed unconscious* – in the real enclave of the unconscious. This means that the imaginary space is interspersed with splinters, capsules, or crypts, consisting of neither translatable nor transformable beta sensations. These "objects a" are gathered in the form of splinters on or in the beta-screen and are stabilized there by the early defensive form of splitting, i.e., more or less solidly removed from the rest of the psychic world as mini-enclaves of the real unconscious. The asymbolic pole I is located in area B (cf. Figure 10.1). If the individual experiences an internal or external crisis, the critical moments (e.g., consisting of relationship conflicts, experiences of loss) act as triggers that release the real beta sensations isolated in the form of stimulus protection. They spread throughout the body, dissipate in behavior (*passage à l'acte*), or are transferred onto the object – the Other – via projective identification. Marty (1968) describes the formation of physical symptoms as the result of a "reversible" or "regressive" somatization.

Temporary complaints may occur, such as headaches from muscular tension, fluctuations in blood pressure, diarrhea, constipation, upper abdominal discomfort, and complaints resulting from the stimulation of specific centers in the brain, such as pain centers (cf. Stora, 2007, p. 38).

Another pole, the asymbolic pole II, localized on a vertical axis, concerns psychosomatically precipitated severe physical illnesses. That is where advancing, i.e., progressive, somatization takes place, which may even lead to lethal physical diseases, such as a heart attack, via a material organ lesion (e.g., inflammation and calcification of the coronary vessels). And that is where the imaginary space is severely damaged: Riddled with multiple beta-splinters, it is transformed into something empty and desolate that manifests in the atmosphere of "essential depression" (Marty, 1968; Stora, 2007, p. 38). Real sensations are split off or rejected altogether. However, if real sensations are triggered and released, their sheer force leads to lesions in the physical organs which are particularly vulnerable because of additional physical or genetic risk factors. The intensity of the split-off sensation, the devastation of the imaginary space, the traumatic quality of the trigger, and the physical vulnerability are the factors that determine the course of "progressive" somatization in the context of a "progressive disorganization."

Hypochondria may be localized at the logical pole, at the opposite side of a somatological, vertical vector, now a mental phenomenon that can be both symbolic (conversion neurotic, hysterical) and asymbolic (operative). In any case, hypochondria belongs to area A (cf. Figure 10.2) as part of the imaginary–symbolic, i.e., mental, conceptions about the body based on alpha elements.

At the center of the psychosomatic, imaginary space lies the imaginary zone, where the real, the imaginary, and the symbolic are in intimate contact with one another and are not compromised by strong defenses. The real sensation neither has to be repressed nor split off nor foreclosed. It is a bodily experience that one can understand as a symptomatic response to a situation or the message of the Other (cf. Morel, 2019 [2008]), for instance, in the form of a scream, a fall, a plunge, or some form of tension, freezing, cold, or horror. But by not having to mobilize any substantial defense, the imaginary remains in atmospheric experiential proximity to the real. The real thing of sensation (in area B, see Figure 10.2) can be translated as a bodily feeling, i.e., determined imaginarily and symbolically (in area A), without the need for splitting off (area B) or repression (area A, see Figure 10.2).

That is the theoretical model, which is intended to have a logical consistency and, in the Euclidean tradition, to represent the creative compilation and systematization of psychoanalytic knowledge about the reciprocal relationship between body and mind. This systematization takes place in the sense of the "king's sciences." Yet psychoanalytic practice, as we shall see, is more akin to nomadic thinking, where the map is reinvented each time, just as sailors who set out into the open sea to discover new continents harbor certain ideas about the spherical or disc-shaped nature of the world. Psychoanalytic practice means undertaking nomadic forays into the unconscious, which is enclosed or repressed.

Expeditions and Travel Stories

The first story reports a journey or an expedition into the imaginary zone. Georg has come to see me because he has been suffering for weeks from conditions of near paralysis. Indeed, he then proceeds to lie on his sofa without moving, mentally or physically. He feels nothing, cannot get up, cannot speak or think, and is no longer present at all. The EMS had to be called several times. Everyone stands around him, looking at him helplessly.

The only affect he feels is a huge, worrying fear that, as he later reports, knows no bounds. During this time, he worries a lot and is often suddenly tormented and desperate because he does not know what is wrong with him and why he continues to fall into such paralyzing pits. For example, once, during a garden party at Georg's home, everyone else – his neighbors, friends, and some colleagues from the sports club – is quite cheerful and relaxed. The weather is nice, etc. Georg, although considered a rather shy, sophisticated type, is quite popular and clearly integrated in this down-to-earth world of single-family homes and garden plots – just outside a medium-sized Swiss town. He is quite successful as a real estate agent. But, this afternoon, he feels numb, disconnected, and set apart from everything. This separateness exhausts him makes him feel powerless, so suddenly he has to withdraw from the party noise and the relaxed affability of his guests. Nothing seems to work anymore. He begins to tremble inside, has tinnitus, has to lie down, feels weak, and has a headache.

Up to that time, Georg's whole disastrous childhood had not played a role in his present life. He had simply blanked it out, forgotten it, and locked everyone from earlier out of his personal life. Only during analysis, because I have become interested in it, does he begin to tell the harrowing story of his childhood. It is one of poverty, violence, chaos, powerlessness, shame, disorientation, suffering, and alcohol. The father was an alcoholic, a giant of a man, a grim, rough-hewn hulk (or so Georg remembers) who was always drunk when he showed up at home, always irritable and frustrated. With seven children and an utterly overburdened wife, who came across as a pale, fearful woman torn between violence and poverty, this father, who himself felt inwardly lost, always found reason to be irritated, indignant, and upset. Once, in a gesture of neglect (little Georg was also present), his older brothers had set fire to a wooden hut. The boys then squatted in a tree until late at night to avoid being beaten half to death by their father. Returning home was always terrible for them because you could only sneak in crouched down, with the father standing in the front door. He often beat the mother, who would then disappear for days, so the children had to fend for themselves. (I would like to skip the external causes, the violent relationship conflict with all the abandonment, disappointments, and verbal violence, and jump to speaking about the following session.)

In one session during the second year of the analysis, Georg loses his grip completely. The bodily feeling does not arise suddenly, but it seems to me, gradually: like an inner decline, a slip-sliding that prevents him from speaking; he falls silent, becomes still, and begins to fall. As his analyst, I am present and attentive, and it wouldn't surprise me if I lean forward a bit. But I don't say anything, I don't try to interrupt this falling (i.e., the falling process) with anything. The emotional atmosphere in the room is that I am *there*: It is a "space of experienced presence" filled with the atmosphere of a feeling (Schmitz, 2020, p. 34). Perhaps one can portray this with an image of an archway or a door that turns into an entrance to the labyrinth of the rhizome. Georg now speaks, somewhat quietly and soberly, as he always does:

Georg: "I'm just falling ..."

The atmosphere is such that we share the space of our feelings, that is, our feelings are present in the imaginary space of the treatment room, expanding in this space. My feeling can be described as full of concern, attention, and sympathy; I am affected, but that is not in the foreground, merely present, like a background color. Thus, both Georg's fall and my presence take place within this atmospheric space.

I now go one step further and try to make contact with the bodily sensation of falling or, as one might put it phenomenologically, with Georg's "bodily atmosphere" of falling (Schmitz, 2020, p. 16). If I am to enter into this contact, it helps to surrender all thoughts and notions of control and create an atmospheric or imaginary free space where the feeling of falling can be permitted. Husserl (1999 [1907], p. 23) speaks of the attitude of the *epoché,* which, anchored in this free space, allows an unreserved contemplation of an object, of just such a feeling. This is not about dissecting, analyzing, or reconstructing something but about phenomenal perception. Using this openness, I enter into Georg's falling; I form part of this atmosphere of his bodily feeling, enter the space of this body or bodily life (Schmitz, 2020, p. 16). I enter the outline of the archway, the feeling of falling – allow the bodily feeling of falling to extend to me. I am in this space, and this space is in me. One could, depending on temperament, also speak of a leap into the Imaginary (Ruettner et al., 2015).

The above represent the mere linguistic expressions of a bodily sensation, albeit one that is deeper, more intense, more intimate, and more gripping than what can be put into words.[2] But there are also bodily symptoms that are more or less sealed off; they appear, for example, in the form of a muscular spasm. The material excitement spreads in the body because the real (ideal) sensation cannot be translated and mentalized in any other way, imaginatively or symbolically. Here, the technique of entering is impossible. One feels it immediately; one remains left behind. The decision is an intuitive one: We are in area B (see Figure 10.2), that is, in the enclave of the real unconscious. But the bodily symptoms are symbolic (metaphors) because of a modification of the body image in the repressed unconscious (area A in Figure 10.2). They refer to a repressed unconscious fantasy. The body symbol is more of a sideshow, a distraction from the true desire, the realization of which is made impossible. However, the bodily feeling in the imaginary zone invites us to enter the atmospheric space. So, I allow myself to fall. It is unpleasant: I can't get my footing. It is a fall into wherever, yet I don't know what will come. In any case, I first feel the falling in my chest, which is like a specific island in my body, before the feeling takes hold of the whole body.

I stay with the feeling and don't have to ask Georg to stay with it either – he does it regardless. Otherwise, I would have suggested to him to stay with the bodily feeling (without much or further explanation to avoid distracting from the process). Probably, sooner or later, this bodily feeling would become unbearable. Then it comes to a head, perhaps acquiring the quality of something terrible, threatening, and exposed. That the fall accelerates, that fear rises, that all contact is lost – that's where the danger lies, typical for such a situation, of falling into the real, i.e., the bodily feeling loses its imaginary constitution, and something nonrepresented or nonrepresentable derived from early traumas gains the upper hand. In this respect, the bodily feeling is indeed a "superficial abyss" (Baudrillard, 1990 [1979], p. 53): One passes through the imaginary surface of the symptom into the abyss of real sensations. You must suffer through this real state, at least for a while. This situational breakdown is possible only because it occurs in the emotional atmosphere of being carried. Nonetheless, the transference (or the analyst's factual behavior allied to the transference) may contain an essential, albeit perhaps subtle, trigger. Lacan's sketch shows this moment of transgression into the real.

In Figure 10.4, the green line (the imaginary) crosses over into the red line of the real. But what is unbearable – the hopelessness of falling, the touching of the real – is the validation of the imaginary bodily feeling. Lacan represented these processes graphically as shown in Figure 10.4 (Lacan, 1976–1977, p. 81).

The unbearable, i.e., the touching of the real, is the validation of the imaginary bodily feeling. To save themselves, sooner or later, either the analysts or the analysands as it were pulled the ripcord of symbolization – the

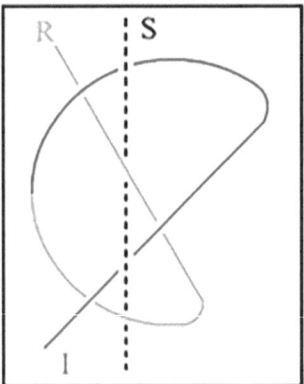

Figure 10.4 The relation of the real, the imaginary, and the symbolic in the zone of the imaginary (cf. Lacan, 1976–1977, p. 81). This illustration was taken from the French edition, Staferla version.

blue line in Figure 10.4. de M'Uzan (1989) describes a similar protective measure to prevent the analyst from becoming psychotic. This symbolization, whether utilizing inner images (still in the imaginary register) or employing language (already in the symbolic register), is a response to the real: It serves as an emergency brake or a parachute. Symbolization begins when one allows images to emerge while falling, providing a secure foothold: The symbolic parachute opens. This scene is an imaginary translation of the sensation of falling, whereas the actual fall, something we call "being dropped," remains hidden in the real. Here, we are dealing not (only) with the (subsequent) reconstruction of a traumatic scene, namely, that the mother is beaten, but also with a deeper experience in which words function as placeholders, including everything quoted in this chapter.

I see a woman looking away, in half-profile, against a white (or blank) background. The image is somewhat stylized, perhaps like a Marc Chagall painting; I associate his art with youth, floating love, loss, and homesickness for Vitebsk (Chagall's birthplace), which he, the oldest of nine siblings, reinvented in his work. His father worked in a herring depot, his mother ran a small grocery store, etc. – I decide to communicate something to Georg and use the content of the picture because I believe that the imaginary nature of the picture that emerges in me and the imaginary nature of the bodily feeling are atmospherically closer to each other than if I had offered a more abstract interpretation. To keep my communication open and accessible, I don't say, "A woman is looking away," but rather:

Analyst: "Someone is looking away."

My feeling is that these words fit the overall structure of an image ("A woman looks away") and a bodily feeling ("falling"). Any further specification would have been too distracting. So, I search for a balance between defense (toward the real, the incomprehensible) and symbolizing creativity, that is, that Georg and I succeed in taking up a chain of signifiers (S1 – Sn). Symbolization, and with it the rêverie of the analyst, is always both: a defense and a creative transformation. In any case, my sense of falling evaporates, and our path consists of moving in the spaces of the labyrinth, wholly and simply following whatever opens up. This path is labyrinthine, rhizomatic, an interplay of defense and desire that determines the nomadic roaming, moving forward, putting one foot after the other; in other words, the atmospheric ground plan, the language of the labyrinth, the contingent–incontingent sequence or flight of significant spaces. After a while, Georg says:

Georg: "That was … my father hit my mother, I think with an umbrella. He was completely out of control."

I see the image of the father, this giant of a man, hitting Georg's mother, who is half lying on the floor, full of rage. The mother is trying to protect herself with her forearms:

Analyst: "She looked away."
Georg: "No, no, well, yes – but the bad thing was, the terrible thing: *I* looked away! *I* can't watch it, *I* just hear the screaming. He has this umbrella in his hand – and I, I can't do anything, I can't do anything ..."

Silence ensues, we wait. I don't want to decide which experience is deeper or more traumatic: the observation of the (sexual) violence toward the mother who can't hold the child and keeps disappearing from the scene? Or Georg's own helplessness, including his shame at being unable to save the mother? A swarm of signifiers forms: S1, S2, S3 ... – different spaces arising from the fall, open up like a labyrinth. Georg now says:

"I feel really heavy. My hands are totally heavy. I can hardly move them. Everything is so heavy."

The heaviness is the blockage, also the blocked anger. Georg's hands are so heavy that he can't even lift them. Everything is concentrated in that heaviness. Then he says softly:

"Now I'm down."
  "Down where?" I ask.
  "On the couch!" he answers and laughs.

In the subsequent sessions, we work through the feeling of powerlessness, the inner falling, the helplessness, the fear, also the deep shame of being unable to help the mother, the existential fear, the violation of the ego ideal, Oedipus, and the effects of the sadistic superego. Georg manages to put everything into words and share it with me. He begins to recognize the present triggers and to situate them in his history. He becomes more active in his family, clarifying and identifying conflicts. He now experiences the competence he never had as a child. I think his bodily feelings provided access to his traumatic, terrible, violent childhood, which had been buried behind repressions and detachments as well as behind the desire to forget all these terrible things. There must have been some trigger, perhaps an inattention on my part or a sudden memory, that triggered the bodily sensation of falling (or being dropped), and that could be allowed to happen in the safety of our relationship. Thus, the symptoms of the imaginary zone allowed access to a lost time I was able to participate in with the help of bodily-empathic identification and translation.

I want to outline here other routes or paths of psychosomatic symptom formation and the respective interventions, which take place at the symbolic pole, or at the asymbolic pole I.

During her analysis, Anne, a teacher by profession, who grew up in a small town in southern Germany, develops the feeling of a foreign body in her left thigh. It is not really disturbing, but still somewhat irritating to her. She fantasizes that this foreign body rises and falls, depending on how she feels. Yet, perhaps it is the other way around: Maybe she feels good when the foreign body is erect, notices this feeling, only to then feel decrepit, worthless, and weak when the foreign body goes limp or disappears altogether. Occasionally, her legs are so weak that she can hardly walk, and she has to hold onto the edge of the table. We work through the fantasy: From the admired, erotic, and attractive father who resembles a movie star and possesses a phallus (or a baby), to the fear of the envious, cold mother whom she would have preferred to be rid of. Of course, we could have delved into the bodily symptom here as well, since imaginary bodily images are clearly active. But in this case, the bodily symptom is a sideshow, namely, the symbolic representation of unconscious (transference) fantasies (e.g., carrying the phallus of the father/analyst inside, having a baby, being a baby or a phallus). Here, it makes more sense to bring up the latent unconscious and lust, allowing the physical symptoms to subside over time, i.e., by working through the repressed symbolic–imaginary fantasies. So, we explore the (material) symptoms that express a modification of the repressed symbolic–imaginary bodily image (in area A, see Figure 10.2), according to which the enigmatic, seductive, and erotic message of the father was translated but immediately repressed once again, only to manifest itself in the bodily symptom.

A completely different situation appears with patients who live operatively, i.e., who have poor access to their affects, who fantasize little, and whose bodily symptoms – whether in regressive or progressive somatization, as a temporary headache or a heart attack – represent merely a material surface. Here, it is primarily a matter of building an affective-imaginary world before symbols can be understood. Feelings of loneliness, of being lost, of anger, or of hurt must be first discovered and then labeled – in their respective context, from childhood to the present everyday life. Sometimes, it is acceptable if the analyst, upon noting a first inkling of early pains, describes them in babytalk, using the simplest and clearest words, so that the pressure on the body eases with time.

During her analysis, Gerda, a young woman, reported that she had recently experienced back pain again. Gerda had grown up in a family in which feelings were rarely expressed. She experienced her affective inner life – not to speak of sexuality – as something messy, unclean, and in any case irritating. Particularly, her mother functioned at an anal level, excluding all affects. We discovered in the analysis that even feelings of loneliness, sadness, and not being understood were hardly mirrored or processed in the form of containing. Gerda had come to analysis because of physically experienced panic attacks after beginning to ponder the end of her childless marriage. Now Gerda was having back pain again. A friend asked her if she knew the cause of the pain. I asked, "What did you answer?" In response, Gerda said, quietly, almost like a child, speaking more to herself, "It occurs when I feel lonely, even around people." By now, we both knew how this feeling of loneliness as a child ignored by everyone had come about. As mentioned, at the beginning of analysis, she was experiencing only back pain and the physical effects of panic attacks, which appeared in the form of constant regressive somatizations. Over time, Gerda discovered her feelings of loneliness, learned about their causes, and established a notion of their excessive presence in her body, i.e., in her back muscles.

Psychoanalytic–Phenomenological Royal Roads

Deleuze and Guattari (1987) describe the world as a "rhizome," a passageway or tuber-like construction that lies underground or just above the ground. They position this as a counterimage to the metaphor of the tree with its extended root system based on binary branching. The rhizome, on the other hand, is a multirooted, intertwined system:

> A rhizome may be broken, shattered at a given spot, but it will start up again on one of its old lines, or on new lines. (Deleuze & Guattari, 1987, p. 9)

The rhizome reflects heterogeneous elements and connects arbitrary points:

> Every rhizome contains lines of segmentarity according to which it is stratified, territorialized, organized, signified, attributed, etc., as well as lines of deterritorialization down which it constantly flees. (Deleuze & Guattari, 1987, p. 9)

Each point of a rhizome can thus be connected to any other points; the elements are heterogeneous links in a complex chain, decentralized and antihierarchical. The essential elements are not the points but the lines that connect them: Multiplicities grow linearly (Deleuze & Guattari, 1987, p. 9). A rhizome is thus a map:

> The map is open and connectable in all of its dimensions; it is detachable, reversible, susceptible to constant modification. It can be torn, reversed, adapted to any kind of mounting, reworked by an individual, group, or social formation. It can be drawn on a wall, conceived of as a work of art, constructed as a political action or as a meditation. Perhaps one of the most important characteristics of the rhizome is that it always has multiple entryways. (Deleuze & Guattari, 1987, p. 12)

One such entrance is the bodily symptom, located in the imaginary zone. The "royal road" here means abandoning oneself to the path of the bodily sensation – such as falling or tinnitus, back pain, coldness in the bones, or itching – and following this path, which is unpredictable: From the moment of the first perception of the bodily sensation to some other point, which may be located in real life, in the enclave of the unconscious. From there, further lines lead through the sections, layers, and segments of the imaginary and the symbolic. One can follow these intuitively, without knowing in advance where the path leads, either with an attitude of *epoché* or, as Bion says, by renouncing more specific desires or specific knowledge. This is true even if here, in this labyrinth, we do follow a desire, even if it contains the – incestuous – desire to enter such a labyrinth. The symbolization is Ariadne's thread that leads out again after having encountered the "Minotaur of the Real." Here, we experience the difference between perception and a symbolically, i.e., linguistically, composed interpretation. The latter is a kind of transformative meditation on the real sensation triggered by a perception.

Another entranceway for rhizomatic work is the dream, a slip of the tongue, a "Freudian blunder," a narrative. But asymbolic, operative bodily symptoms are also entryways, although they may lead nowhere: They are dead ends, and we must first build the labyrinth that serves as a home for the "Minotaur of the Real." Here, the main thing is to construct a phenomenal, felt world that can be determined imaginatively, symbolically, pictorially, and linguistically. At the symbolic pole, on the other hand, it seems important to engage with those lines that lead into the chambers of the unconscious imagination, the repressed unconscious, and not exclusively follow the lines of bodily sensation. Deleuze and Guattari write in this regard:

> The map has to do with performance, whereas the tracing always involves an alleged "competence." Unlike psychoanalysis, psychoanalytic competence (which confines every desire and statement to a genetic axis or overcoding structure, and makes infinite, monotonous tracings of the stages on that axis or the constituents of that structure), schizoanalysis rejects any idea of pretraced destiny, whatever name is given to it—divine, anagogic, historical, economic, structural, hereditary, or syntagmatic. (Deleuze & Guattari, 1987, p. 12 f.)

I think we are dealing here with a dialectic of the copy (in the sense of reproduction, repetition, iteration) and the map (in the sense of following, roaming, wandering, and intineration) (cf. Wendt, 2015). The "model of psychic relations" and the related "axis of psychosomatic totality" are blueprints of the labyrinth, just as labyrinths are depicted on Cretan coins, for example

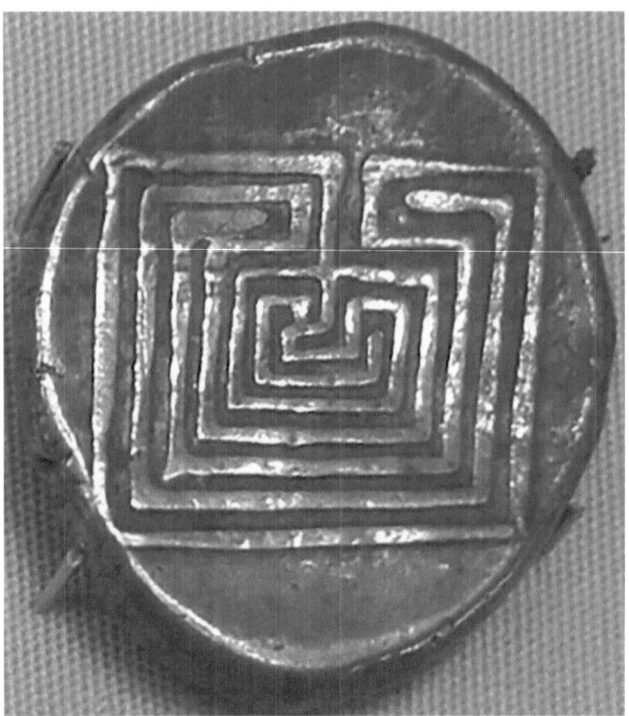

Figure 10.5 The labyrinth on a silver coin from Knossos, 400 B.C. (https://commons. wikimedia.org/wiki/File:Knossos_silver_coin_400bc.jpg).

(Figure 10.5). I believe these blueprints help assess the entrances into the labyrinth, i.e., to some extent the bodily symptoms, to know where one stands at all, how to, as Deleuze and Guattari (1987, p. 14) say, "make a rhizome".

Within the rhizome, however, only nomadic roaming is possible. Leave aside the analytic copy, forget the coin in hand, put it in brackets, and rely entirely on the "performance of cartography." An (analytical) copy always "amounts to the same thing." The map, on the other hand, evolves during the session, its elements establishing themselves as "plateaus," as points of connection, as situational links (Deleuze & Guattari, 1987, p. 21): The fall is a plateau, as is the sofa, the phallus erection, and the back pain. We make the lines and connections by following these links intuitively. Thus, the "royal road" of the model, the copy, the princely mirror, and the royal science are transformed into nomadic paths, roaming through the atmosphere of the unconscious: The intertwining of both sciences – of royal theory and nomadic practice – that is what gives psychoanalysis its special charm.

Notes

1 Wolff (1992, p. 46) explains this passage to denote "ideality" (or "ideational") when something "exists only for the point of view or in the perspective of a particular observer." Ideational means being available only to a particular observer. Wolff thinks this beholder can only be an individual human being. Hegel, however, does not speak of a beholder but of a "theoretical process" or of the "standpoints of sensation" from which the immaterial part of materiality can be perceived (both from the point of view of the other and of self-reflection).
2 Schmitz (2020, p. 19) differentiates the spatiality of emotional and bodily atmospheres (bodily feelings): The former are extended in space or absolute, the latter more local or partial. Thus, the local (partial) bodily feeling of falling is embedded in the more extended emotional atmosphere of attentiveness and presence.

References

Baudrillard, J. (1990 [1979]): *Seduction*. Trans. by B. Singer. Montreal: New World Perspectives.
Bion, W. R. (1962): *Learning from Experience*. London: Tavistock.
Dejours, C. (2001): *Le corps d'abord – Corps biologique, Corps érotique et sens moral*. Paris: Payot.
Deleuze, G. & Guattari, F. (1987 [1976]): *A Thousand Plateaus*. Trans. by B. Massumi. Minneapolis – London: Minnesota Press.
Demmerling, C. (2021): Gefühle und der begriffliche Raum des menschlichen Lebens. *Dt Z Philos*, 69, 347–364.
Evans, D. (1996): *An Introductory Dictionary of Lacanian Psychoanalysis*. London – New York: Routledge.
Freud, S. (1900): *The Interpretation of Dreams*. SE IV, ix–627.
Goetzmann, L. (2020): Gamma elements as protomental representations: Suggestions for expanding W. R. Bion's model of elements. *Int J Psychoanal*, 101, 1085–1105. 10.1080/00207578.2020.1822145
Goetzmann, L., Siegel, A. & Ruettner, B. (2020): On the axis of psychosomatic totality. *Eur J Psychoanal*. Online: https://www.journal-psychoanalysis.eu/on-the-axis-ofpsychosomatic-totality/ [retrieved on 3 November 2021].
Hamburger, A. (2013): Via Regia und zurück. Traumerzählungen und ihre Resonanz. In: Janta, B., Unruh, B. & Walz-Pawlita, S. (Eds.): *Der Traum*. Gießen: Psychosozial, 123–143.
Hegel, G. W. F. (2010 [1830]): *Encyclopedia of the Philosophical Sciences. Part I: Science of Logic*. Cambridge: Cambridge University Press.
Husserl, E. (1999 [1907]): *The Idea of Phenomenology*. Trans. by L. Hardy. Collected Works, Vol. VIII; Dordrecht-Boston-London: Kluver Publishers.
Kluge, A. & Vogl, J. (2009): Was ist ein Rhizom? In: Kluge, A. & Vogl, J.: *Soll und Haben*. Zürich: Diaphanes, 309–320.
Lacan, J. (1976–1977): L'insu que sait de l'une-bévue s'aile à mourre. Online: http://staferla.free.fr/S24/S24%20L%27INSU ... .pdf [retrieved on 24 November 2021].
Lacan, J. (2016 [1962/63]): *Anxiety. The Seminar of Jacques Lacan. Book X*. Cambridge: Polity Press.
Lacan, J. (2021 [1974–1975]). R.S.I. The Seminar of Jacques Lacan, Book XXII. Lacan in Ireland, http://www.lacaninireland.com/web/wp-content/uploads/2010/06/RSI-Complete-With-Diagrams.pdf.

Laplanche, J. (1999). Notes on afterwardness. In: Fletcher, J. (Ed.): *Essays on Otherness*. London: Routledge, pp. 260–265.

Laplanche, J. (2004): Die rätselhaften Botschaften des Anderen und ihre Konsequenzen für den Begriff des Unbewussten im Rahmen der Allgemeinen Verführungstheorie. *Psyche – Z Psychoanal*, 58, 898–913.

Laplanche, J. (2011). *Freud and the Sexual*. London: Karnac.

Marty, P. (1968): A major process of somatization: The progressive disorganization. *Int J Psychoanal.*, 49, 246–249.

Morel, G. (2019 [2008]): *The law of the mother. An essay on the sexual sinthome*. London: Routledge.

Rau-Luberichs, D. (2016): Wenn der Körper "spricht." Der bewegte Körper als neuer Königsweg in der psychodynamischen Psychotherapie. In: Gödde, G. & Stehle, S. (Eds.): *Die therapeutische Beziehung in der psychodynamischen Psychotherapie*. Gießen: Psychosozial, 313–338.

Ruettner, B., Siegel, A., & Goetzmann, L. (2015): Der Sprung ins Imaginäre – zur Behandlungstechnik im Umgang mit Körpersymptomen. *Psyche – Z Psychoanal*, 8, 714–736.

Sami-Ali, M. (2006): *Penser le somatique. Imaginaire et pathologie*. Paris: Dunod.

Schmitz, H. (2011): *Der Leib*. Berlin/Boston: de Gruyter.

Schmitz, H. (2020): *Atmosphären. Freiburg/München*: Karl Aber.

Stora, J. B. (2007): *When the body displaces the mind*. London: Karnac.

Wendt, D. (2015): Narrativer Nomadismus. Raum und Wissen bei Herodot (im Anschluss an Deleuze). etopoi. *Journal for Ancient Studies*, 5, 86–109.

Wolff, M. (1992): *Das Körper-Seele-Problem*. Kommentar zur Hegel, Enzyklopädie (1830), § 369. Frankfurt a. M.: Vittorio Klostermann.

de M'Uzan, M. (1989): Während der Sitzung – Überlegungen zum psychischen Geschehen im Analytiker. *Jahrbuch für Psychoanalyse*, 31, 77–99.

Žižek, S. (2007): *The Indivisible Remainder. On Schelling and Related Matters*. London – New York: Verso.

Chapter 11

Mentalized Alterity
Psychodynamic Work with Bodily Countertransference

Timo Storck

Introduction: Links to the Body in Psychosomatics

From a clinical perspective, we can describe the psychodynamics of the body by resorting to three levels of friction and (seemingly) paradox: the level of symptoms, the level of psychodynamic conflict, and the level of resonance.

Symptomatically, there is a tension between an apparent mental void, in terms of being emptied out of emotional vitality, and some sort of somatic "chaos," with a body that is burdened, aching, or dysfunctional. At first glance, these seem to be two different, distinct kinds of symptoms, yet I shall later come back to the conceptual notion that they can be traced back to a common factor underlying them.

On the level of psychodynamic conflict, we can speak of a tension between the dynamics of disconnection and the dynamics of fusion. On the one hand, this is about psyche and soma appearing as not being connected to one another. Mental life appears to stand in opposition to an objectified body that is being perceived from a distance, being repelled, or solely experienced as a source of pain – the mental and the somatic are not linked in an integral relation. On the other hand, we can describe the phenomena of experiencing fusion, wherein boundaries or outlines are missing or unstable (which is also the case regarding object relations to personal others).

Third, we can include a level of resonance, and this points to the experience of emotional distance and detachment that presents itself in clinical work. A patient appears "far away" from us, or we feel a huge emotional distance between them and us. At the same time, however, we experience a "pressure toward identity" within the analytic relationship which will be described in more detail later, a pull toward sameness or completion.

I shall further explore all three levels (mental void opposed to somatic chaos, disconnection opposed to fusion, distance opposed to pressure toward identity) and trace them back to an underlying impaired capacity to tolerate otherness which manifests on a psychosomatic level. I shall then elaborate on these notions toward some implications and proposals for treatment techniques. These will be summed up as "mentalized alterity" which strives

DOI: 10.4324/9781003370130-11

for representing the other's otherness while being related. In order to do this, embracing the co-created bodily experience within the analytic relationship will turn out to be the most important cornerstone.

Some of the thoughts on psychosomatic theories and views on the body in psychoanalysis presented here can be also found in previous works (Storck, 2016a,b; Storck, 2020a; Storck & Brauner, 2021).[1]

Conceptual Background

First, some conceptual clarifications need to be made. As mentioned in the title, the thoughts presented here are related to "psychodynamic work with bodily countertransference" – what do we mean by "bodily," "counter-transference," and "psychodynamic work?"

In the following, I will base my ideas on the way philosophical anthropology or phenomenology commonly use "having a body" (Körper) and "being a body" (Leib) (cf. Kobylinska-Dehe, 2019). This goes back to Hellmuth Plessner (see also Alloa et al., 2012). This distinction places the human body we "have" on the physical level – this "body" is which we can weigh or measure in other ways, the one that aches if we bruise our arm or the one we accelerate when sprinting to reach the bus that is already driving off. While the body we "have" is the object of perception, volition, and so on, the body we "are" can be understood on the level of experience and its modalities. In this, the body is not just a tool for perception but the very subject of experience, a "functioning" (fungierend) body in a Husserlian sense which represents its own conditions of possibility of relating to the world. When sprinting to reach the bus, the body we have is set into motion, whereas bodily (by means of the body we are) we feel how the airflow feels while sprinting. The body we *have* is an object of our experience, whereas the body we *are* is a felt experience from the perspective of a subjective body which changes as soon as we try and make it the object of our thoughts. The difference presents itself most prominently in the field of "psychosomatic" symptoms in a clinical sense: In pathogenesis, the body that is aching or impaired in its functions has become a mere body one has, it has lost the quality of a body one is – with the result that one strives to get rid of it or have it operated. Also, we should note that usually we are able to shift perspectives between viewing the body we are and the body we have (Fuchs, 2015; Küchenhoff, 2012): We shift between an object perspective on the body we have and a subject perspective arising from the body we are, the latter being understood as an experiential form of wholeness and permeability between psyche and soma. A similar notion can be found in Leikert's (2019) thoughts on the bodily self and encapsulated kinetic engrams. The author views those engrams as "devitalized somatic configurations" (p. 27) or "sealed schemata" (p. 86). Leikert conceives of processes of inhibition and dissocia-tion as a form of "kinetic defence" that leads to the bodily self (as a way of "self-perception mediated through the body"; p. 64) and the body memory not being connected with other systems of experience and memory. Rather, an "isolated configuration" (p. 93) persists. The bodily self as well as the mental cathexis of representational systems are paralyzed (see below for consequences for treatment technique).

Furthermore, the concept of countertransference deserves a brief review. In line with several other authors, I differentiate on a conceptual level, not an experiential one, between the analyst's countertransference and his or her own transference (Storck, 2020b). Countertransference then can be understood as that part of the therapist's experience which stems from the dynamics of the encounter with a patient. Traditionally, this has been described as some sort of response to the patient's transference. Yet, there have been comments on how what happens in the clinical situation can hardly be seen as linear sequences of transference and countertransference where the latter follows the former logically or temporally. Nevertheless, we can propose that something on the analyst's side has to do with the fact that he or she is talking with that very person in that very moment. In the face of the analytic stance, we give special regard to how a patient uses the relational offer to deploy himself or herself both consciously and unconsciously. Thus, it is not by chance that the focus is on the patient's contribution to the analytic relationship. The analyst's own transference then can be understood as those aspects of his or her experience that show themselves in a treatment or single session independently from the patient – as something the analyst brings to the treatment or session independently from the particular relational dynamics. For example, the therapist might feel tense because of a private phone call he or she received right before the start of the session. Obviously, this is a mere abstract, conceptual differentiation; of course, both (the analyst's countertransference and transference) come together in each moment of clinical work, and a huge part of the art of psychoanalysis consists of reflecting both in order to give sound and helpful interpretations. I tried to grasp this challenge by resorting to the image of a "countertransference jukebox." Like with a song you cannot seem to get out of your head (in German: an "earworm"), an analyst brings something utmost personal into his or her view on what happens in a session, yet this can be understood as a form of being resonant with the tone of the session, which is set by a patient (Storck, 2021d).

Finally, some remarks on "psychodynamic work" will prove to be helpful. In the following, I will write about thoughts on those forms of psycho-therapeutic treatment that build on psychoanalytic theory and treatment techniques. The scope of what follows should not be restricted to an unmodified high-dose psychoanalysis using the couch setting. However, one should highlight that the basic analytical rules, such as free association and evenly suspended attention, as well as the fostering of regression and working through the countertransference (especially crises and breakdown) can provide a "microscopical" view on bodily dynamics. These show themselves more clearly within the traditional psychoanalytic setting. This is not to say, however, that bodily dynamics (in terms of the body we are) and the work regarding them would not play a role in other psychodynamics settings. Also, I will restrict my thoughts in the following to therapeutic conversation; even though (verbal) interventions can hardly be detached from the body, I will not put emphasis on actual interventions in physical therapy or the actual use of the body for therapeutic work.

Being Cut Off from One's Own "Drive Base"

In Freud's work, there is plenty of "being a body" (see Scharff, 2010, regarding the "bodily dimension" in psychoanalysis). This is the case regarding the foundations of drive theory or infantile sexuality from the beginnings of psychoanalytic theory formation. Further, we cannot over-estimate the importance of the notion that within the couch setting motor activity (and thus motor discharge) is prevented so that drive impulses can mediate into fantasies and associations (Freud, 1900, pp. 338, 567). Also, we aim to understand what shows itself symptomatically "in" the body. This stands in opposition to Freud's skepticism toward the possibility of treating so-called "actual neuroses" (as precursors of "somatic symptom disorder" or other terms to describe and classify psychosomatic disorders) psychoanaly-tically: Freud proposed a lacking impact of infantile sexuality and therefore conflict-related etiology in actual neuroses (hypochondria, neurasthenia, and anxiety neurosis) and, as a consequence, a lack of transference processes. Instead of psychoanalytic treatment (promoting insight into unconscious conflictual meaning), there was, according to Freud, rather the need for psychoeducation in terms of sexual life to relieve someone of symptoms of actual neurosis (see Freud, 1916/17, p. 387ff.).

Of course, there have been further developments, first and foremost regarding the conceptualization of bodily symptoms stemming, at least partially, from mental processes but also in terms of a widening scope of indication for psychoanalytic treatment and therefore treatment technique. Among those conceptual developments are ways to describe phenomena that present themselves in the therapeutic relationship, such as operational thinking (Marty & de M'Uzan, 1963) or alexithymia, which play an important role in psychosomatic disorders. Both concepts refer to a mental structure or style of cognition, affect, and communication; they are based on what shows clinically: a way of using language that appears to be "de-subjectified," social over-adaptation, duplication of actions in words (instead of language as a means to add the sphere of experience), or an impression of boredom on the therapist's side while listening to a patient (see von Rad, 1983). Further contributions from the so-called Paris School of Psychosomatics deepen these observations. Marty (1968) develops the notion of an essential depression and, in this, links the somatic symptoms that stem from mental processes to the experience of mental void and being emptied out of affect or sensuality. This kind of depression basically is due to mental experience lacking the permeation by the body one is. It is those patients who get depressed that merely have a body instead of being a body. Aisenstein (2006) or Smadja (2001) conceive of a two-fold group of symptoms: Mental void and the burden of somatic symptoms are connected because both can be traced back to a disruption in the permeation of psyche and soma leading to both being disconnected from one another.

Similar thoughts have been published by Fain (1971) who discusses how auto-erotism, that is, the satisfactory exploration of the body one has and is and the parent attending to it, is pivotal for the development of fantasy life (same as, in more general terms, for a rich, sensual, and emotional inner world). Mcdougall (1978, p. 358) links psychosomatic disorders to the phenomenon of being cut off from one's own "drive base." Psychodynamically, this can be described as a drive pathology. "Drive" can be understood as a concept referring to a mediating function between vegetative states or processes and the level of mental experience (Storck, 2018a). Then, we can also describe how a disruption in the drive-like mediation leads to a loss of the "incentive" which lets mental life progress by means of represented states (which can also be captured by the concept of unconscious fantasy as described by Klein or Isaacs, 1948, as well as by Bion's thoughts on alpha function; Bion, 1962). Also, the body one merely has and no longer is (by way of the disruption of drive-like mediation) has to deal with states of excitation on its own, without mental modulation or representation.

Thus, we arrive at the image of a disconnection between psyche and soma. The individual has become a "dividual." This has been laid out clearly by Lombardi (see, e.g., Karacaoglan & Lombardi, 2018), and we can spot the Aristotelian spark in it: If indeed the soul is the form of the body then both are lost if permeation between the two is suspended.

Also, we can find here a more detailed, "psycho-economical" (i.e., one that refers to mediation through the drive) description and conceptualization of one side of the three levels of tension mentioned at the beginning: the psychodynamics of disconnection, the interpersonal impression of great emotional distance, and symptoms that bring together mental void and somatic chaos. I already shed some light on the last one of those three levels: What I coined "drive pathology" is what makes both kinds of symptoms come about. The other two levels, disconnection in relation to fusion and emotional distance in relation to "identity pressure" are to be elucidated further, regarding the role of the object.

Fusion without Intimacy

Psychoanalytic theories of the body (one is) usually highlight two aspects. The first I just discussed: The mediation and permeation between psyche and soma (this way of describing it already bears the danger of obscuring the fact that psyche and soma do not stand in a pre-set relation of separation or opposition). The other aspect is an object-relational one. Here we can also find a long conceptual history with landmarks such as Anna Freud's (1952, p. 1273) remark on the hypochondriac playing "mother-and-child" with his or her own body (which means: A patient experiences and treats the own body alongside ambivalent wishes of being cared for). Other theories also relate the representation of the body and object representation to one another (see Plassmann, 1993, for "organ worlds" in that regard). One particular way of conceptualizing this can be seen in Mcdougall's (1989, p. 25) notion of "one body for two" (see also Kutter, 2001, for a "fighting over the body").

Two elements stick out here. One, the dynamics of a superimposition, fusion, or inseparation of representations of one's own body and that of the personal other. In a very concrete sense, the aching or dysfunctional body one has can be seen as the incorporation of an ambivalent interpersonal relationship in which there is no one with or without the other. In this, the symptom serves as an "index" (Küchenhoff, 2019), pointing broadly to the fact that there is something conflictual in relationships which, on the most fundamental level, has to do with the regulation of intimacy and distance. Second, related to that, there is the dynamics of a (torturing, yet life-saving) dependency on a "key person" (Engel & Schmale, 1967). There is an urge for the actual presence of a helpful other, in a symbiotic partnership or family relation, or in contacting medical and/or psychotherapeutic care. In this strong urge for the presence of the other, it appears to be interchangeable who serves this function of an envisioned completion. Conceptually, this can be traced back to the thought that within this object relation to a key person, it is not the deepened relation of true intimacy but rather, in the words of self-psychology (see, e.g., Kohut, 1984), the basic self-object-relation in which the personal object is needed for the function it serves, which is keeping the (bodily) self intact or complete.

Here, it appears to be important whether and, if so, how the individual can resort to the other to "use" him in a Winnicottian sense: Such an appeal for care (also in a sense of regulation) that is expressed is, if not taken up by a resonant other, what can later be seen in the way a person deals with symptoms. Then, the symptom can serve the function of an appeal to the other (as can be seen in the need for medical checkups) in order to unconsciously involve him in a repetitive, enmeshed mis-en-scène of relational patterns (which can play a prominent role in personality disorders) or keep him within a safe distance (in a pattern of bodily distance).

These are the dynamics of fusion on the level of mental representation. One's own body and personal objects lack demarcations in the representational world. Also, regarding object relations, we can generally see that the relation between (bodily) self and object is marked by a specific mode of linkage or fusion. On the level of symptoms, the over-adaptiveness can be traced back to that. If the personal other is needed to feel complete or in unison, this results in the "pressure for identity" mentioned earlier. The individual feels that one has to be similar (or, at least, a complementary fit) in order to make feeling related to one another arise and persist. However, this is not an intimate relationship but a relational mode of imitation or assimilation, either of the self toward the object or of the object toward the self (de M'Uzan, 1977, coined this "projective reduplication").

From this originates a massive intolerance for separation. Being separated (or different from the other) is experienced as if parts of the body that are needed for survival were lost.

We should further take into account that the dynamics of fusion might reduce anxiety (since it appears to allow to feel safe and complete), and it fulfills longings for closeness in a symbiotic mode, yet it is marked by a deep ambivalence: In being as close to the other as in a complete lack of distance or difference, there is a danger of losing the self. It is a kind of fusion with something painful, destructive, or torturing. In other words: The loss of boundaries and limits in a fusion between psyche and soma as well as between self and other promotes helpless attempts to eventually set some kind of boundary or demarcation.

If this is done in a dysfunctional way, psychosomatic symptoms develop and show themselves in the way of relating to others (e.g., in the analytic relationship). Küchenhoff (2010) describes the negativity of symptoms in this regard: Where a non-relation (manifesting itself through the interpersonal impression of emotional distance or boredom on the clinician's side), non-meaning (rejection of emotional significance), or non-cathexis (emotional void) continues to appear, this might be understood as a "no" which is the symptom's function: It is a "no" toward a deepening of the relation to the other because it is feared as a danger to the self. It is a "no" in terms of setting a boundary or demarcation, a substantial repudiation as an attempt to be able to demarcate, separate, and feel different. What this can only bring about, however, is some sort of pseudo-boundary that is not permeable and should be regarded rather as a wall between self and other (see also Leikert, 2021, for the concept of encapsulated bodily engrams).

The lack of boundaries and the search for limits allow us to bring together two levels that have been discussed so far, the "psycho-economical" and the "object-logical" one. The disconnection between psyche and soma (coined above as being cut off from one's own drive base) means setting a boundary through disruption. There is no permeability or formation. The fusion between psyche and soma, between self and other, first and foremost imposes as a lack of boundaries, yet it further calls for a desperate attempt to secure personal coherence by setting an impermeable pseudo-boundary.

This is the dynamics of a primary inflexible border (between psyche and soma) on the one hand and the dynamics of a primary lack of boundaries on the other hand, both responding to one another and trying to defend against the other. Now, both can be linked conceptually by resorting to the axial model proposed by Ferrari (2004).

Dot, Line, Relationship – Unfolding and Compromising the Mental and Social World

A fundamental conceptual relation between (lived) self, body, and personal other can already be found in an often quoted remark by Freud (1923, p. 26). There, he states that the Ego was "first and foremost a bodily Ego," something like the "projection of a surface," stemming from bodily sensations (note that this relates to the body one is and to the body as part of an interpersonal situation of bodily interaction, like in Merleau-Ponty's term of "intercorporeité"; 1964; for its role in developmental psychology and in psychotherapy, see Fuchs, 2003; Broschmann & Fuchs, 2020; for a psychoanalytical perspective, see Kobylinska-Dehe, 2019; Scharff, 2021). In short, this deals with how the subjective experience of identity develops. Subjective identity evolves around questions like "Who am I, what is part of me?" as well as "Who am I not?" (while one should take into account, by resorting to philosophical phenomenology, that things are not that simple when it comes to the self and otherness). Subjective experience of identity develops out of endogenuous and exogenuos bodily sensations that give rise to mental images of how "I" am related to the environment. Here, the experience of boundaries and demarcation plays a special role, by means of bodily touch in interpersonal relations (thus, one should specify Freud's statement to "The self is first and foremost an intercorporeal one"). The self (the representation of who one is) as a projection of the body's surface is created out of the experience of bodily touch as sensing contact at a boundary (between one body and an other's body), in exchange with non-touch or interruptions of touch (similar thoughts can be found in Schultz-Venrath, 2021, p. 199). Alongside this, the individual arrives at representing that "I" am touched by someone else. Representing self and object becomes possible if a borderline at which contact (and touch) takes place is internalized. Potentially, this is the kind of boundary that allows permeation and emotional contact in deepened relationships with others (Merleau-Ponty, 1964, coined this "la chair," the flesh).

The boundary between one's own body and the other's body, the borderline between those two, is the precondition for experiencing demarcations and contour of representations and for experiencing self and other as standing in a relation. Self, other, and the bodies of both belong together in a logic of boundaries and a logic of contact.

The axial model which Ferrari (2004) presents for understanding the individual's psychosomatic self-relation, helps to develop this further. The author distinguishes between one axis where psyche and soma (and thus the relation between the two) are located and another axis where the individual and the surrounding (social) world are located. From these two axes, that is, from their relations that can be displayed in the resulting coordinates, a three-dimensional subjective space for experience unfolds (Ferrari calls this "two-fold"). This space is some sort of emergence between what can be displayed on the two axes/dimensions. If someone is situating himself or herself in a dynamic, permeable, yet limit-able relation between psyche and soma and at the same time and in the same way in a relation between himself as an individual and the social environment, a space for experiencing, representing, and shaping relationships and emotions unfolds.

At the same time, we can picture conceptually the consequences of distortions in the relation of the two axes to one another. One axis has an impact on the other. In cases where the relation between psyche and soma is frozen or interrupted, the relation between the individual and the environment is changed as well, because the experiential space for vital relationships and their representation will not unfold in the manner described above. Also, we can see that in cases where the individual relates to the social world (and experiences it) in a borderless way, marked by isolation, the psychosomatic self-relation to the body is in danger of becoming frozen and interrupted; in this case, there won't be any vital way of relating to the world on the grounds of the body one is. Experience remains two-dimensional (Ferrari: "one-fold"), as if experiencing relationships as well as the self-relation were merely an ensemble of flat lines without any links between them. Also, in severe cases, we can see dynamics that can be described through the image of a dot: states of being either completely unrelated or a complete loss of differentiation, where self, body, and the personal other are one and the same.

Ferrari (2004) points out the role and function of a concrete original object (COO) for mental development. Through this, he shows how the relations between the axes described above and their emergent phenomenon of an unfolded space of experience can be fostered or hindered. In his conceptualization (p. 43ff.), the child is confronted with sensory unrest, with stimuli and states of excitation that can stem from relations to a personal other but do not necessarily have to. The COO (to be understood as sort of a merging of physical body, object representation, and the factual personal other) casts a shadow (which refers to Freud's remark concerning the shadow of the object, 1917, p. 249) and thus provides safety and cooling against the heat of unregulated states of excitation. This then makes development and representation possible. Because the COO has both a stimulating and a "cooling" (calming) effect, the axial model can describe the individual's relation to the environment *in relation* to the relation between psyche and soma: The relation between psyche and soma is regulated by how the individual and the environment are linked.

The axial model allows for an exploration of the fields of tension and apparent paradoxa (mental void vs. somatic chaos, disconnection vs. fusion, distance vs. pressure for identity) mentioned earlier by means of resorting to the conceptual notions described here.

The friction between mental void and somatic chaos can be understood as a drive pathology concerning the drive's mediating function – as a result, the mental is separated from the body and emptied out while the body is stripped off of its role as something the individual is and thus bears a heavy burden.

This does not only have an impact on how one experiences relationships with others and lives within them but can be traced back to common roots, as shown in the axial model: The drive pathology accrues from a strained interaction and that in turn accrues from the drive pathology.

The tension between disconnection and fusion can also be depicted in Ferarri's model. This does not lead to a contradiction because the lack of setting limits between self and other is an expression and a result from the fact that during development there hasn't been any experience of touch in a way that would have helped to set up boundaries and demarcations but rather in a neglectful or intrusive way. Something remains disconnected (psyche and soma), and separation (between self and other) is hard to represent.

Finally, regarding the phenomena of huge emotional distance and disconnection in the analytic relationship on the one hand and the pressure for identity on the other hand, we can also say that both are the result of the same dynamics. What appears to be a huge emotional distance is an expression of helpless and dysfunctional attempts to set up a boundary which however only leads to building up an impermeable wall. At the same time, the individual is guided by the fantasy that only mutual assimilation and completion could secure maintaining contact. This however means paying the price that an in-depth relationship between two different individuals becomes impossible. In this way, the pressure toward identity develops as a counterpart to an intensified uncertainty arising whenever being different or separated is sensed.

Next, I shall try to elaborate on that last aspect. The work on making difference more tolerable and letting a relational, experiential space unfold can be achieved through working with somatic countertransference and respective interventions.

Connection and Difference: Somatic Countertransference and the Unfolding of a Relational, Experiential Space in Clinical Work

Assuming that some patients are pressured to assimilate their own way of experiencing to that of others or even to experience themselves as being unseparated from the start, we can resort to some fundamental aspects of psychoanalytic developmental psychology. So far, we can say that the moment-to-moment shifts between being touched and not being touched are a pivotal impulse in developing the capacity for symbolization which, on the most fundamental level, means to envision one's own experience in front of one's own inner eye. To develop this, a "good enough" caregiver (or more than one) is important since it allows to form images/representations of what is momentarily absent from perception and also, in moments of a relative and temporary distance in the first relationship, to find the alternative of a second relationship. In this way, relations become "thinkable" within a "relational web" in which caregivers and significant others can also stand in relation to one another (Storck, 2019).

If these kinds of experience that have to do with triangulation and thus fostering the capacity for symbolization are missing, particular mode of experiencing one's relatedness to others can result. Without sufficient triangulating experiences, the individual remains at a stage of relating to the world in which difference or separatedness from others becomes unbearable. This creates a pressure to not be left alone and feel sameness between the self and the other. Following Theunissen (1977), Mcdougall (1989, p. 44), or Warsitz (2004), I have coined this as a "Störung der Veranderung" (an impaired process of acknowledging and tolerating otherness) (Storck, 2021a). Clinically, this can manifest in a patient feeling threatened as soon as different positions or perspectives between him and the analyst show up.

When following the question of how such an impairment of the process of acknowledging and tolerating otherness can be addressed, we arrive at different aspects of treatment technique.

Level of Listening I: Exploring the Relational Model

The way a patient experiences himself in relation to others is not self-evident and usually harder to detect than it might seem. As soon as we think of the subjective model of being related as something on the level of representation and thus being under the influence of unconscious aspects then it becomes apparent that a mere verbal self-report of that model is impossible. It will most likely only present itself implicitly. In treatments, we meet the objects not the persons – we get to know the *representations* of the father, the mother, and others, the way a patient experiences the relationship to them.

A way to explore a patient's relational model is the methodology that Argelander (1967) or Lorenzer (1970) called "understanding the scene" (*szenisches Verstehen*) (overview in Storck, 2018b). The most direct way to get a picture of how a patient experiences and acts in relationships lies in that very relationship we are part of in the clinical setting. Here, the pressure for identity described above can show itself; e.g., that we as therapists feel the pressure of not representing anything "of our own" or, respectively, directing a patient completely toward being just like us.

In the case of an impairment in acknowledging and tolerating otherness, this means that we should not mistake our image of being related or not being related in a particular relationship for the way a patient experiences that same relationship. Micro-moments of interpersonal difference can be upsetting in a way and to an extent that we do not always see coming, e.g., in a spontaneous remark we as therapists give in terms of not having had the particular experience a patient talks about but nevertheless forming an image when listening to a patient. From the therapist's perspective, this might be seen as a remark to state that we are resonant toward a patient's narrative and inner world, yet from the patient's perspective, it might be perceived as if we had said: "I live in a whole other world than you and thus we will never be able to share anything at all."

Level of Interventions I: Empathy and Perspective

Regarding this mode of experiencing relations and an underlying impairment of acknowledging and tolerating otherness, I have proposed (Storck, 2020a) resorting to a basic form of intervention that includes a concrete verbal statement of our own position from which we empathize with a patient within the mutually created scene. This can mean introducing an intervention by saying, "When I listen to you, I imagine that ..." or by "To me, what you are describing, feels like ... ." Thus, linking empathy with perspective, we mark that we empathize from our own position and form our own images which are nonetheless related to the patient and his or her narrative.

Goals: Working through Otherness

On an abstract level, the goal of such a working through of otherness or establishing the capacity to acknowledge and tolerate otherness is to make difference and separateness more bearable. Thus, we can extend the model through which relationships are experienced in the direction of making it possible to deepen relationships by means of acknowledging interpersonal difference. Being different and separated does not make relating to others impossible but rather provides the ground for intimacy and true encounter. Loosely connected to the notion from developmental psychology of a mentalized affectivity (see Taubner, 2015, p. 58ff.), which refers to the capacity to not be engulfed by one's affects but rather to represent them, we can speak of the goal of a "mentalized alterity" here. This would mean to represent being different when relating to others.

This calls for a brief remark on the role of the body (one is) in mentalization theory and Mentalization-Based Theory (see Taubner, Fonagy & Bateman, 2019). The roots of the "British" mentalization concept, which relies on the idea to think about one's own and other's behavior as being grounded in mental states, lie partly in the so-called Paris School of Psychosomatics' concept of mentalization (Storck, 2021c). In more recent works from mentalization theory there is a focus on "embodied mentalizing" (Luyten & Fonagy, 2020; for a discussion, see Storck & Brauner, 2021). This refers to the perspective of the body one is during the individual's development of a theory of mind. Schultz-Venrath (2021), albeit in a critical view on embodied mentalizing (p. 26), has recently argued for the introduction of an early and autonomous "body-mode" as one of the pre-mentalizing modes (p. 179 f.). He has shown how this and other modes can be understood in relation to the body (p. 207ff.) as well as the clinical implications of a proposed body-mode lying on the basis of the capacity to mentalize.

One key question is how we can help to establish the capacity for a mentalized alterity and make being different in relationships bearable in clinical work. The mere verbalization of different positions might serve to avoid misunderstandings but does hardly suffice to change mental structures of how one experiences being related to others. Put in Ferrari's model: In cases with psycho-logical conditions marked by overlay and fusion between psyche and soma and individual and social environment that render relational life two- or one-dimensional – what is the means to let mental space for experiencing relations unfold?

Level of Listening II: Phenomena of Somatic Countertransference

Conceptualizing countertransference has covered some distance in the history of psychoanalysis, at times touching upon ethical aspects of psychotherapy and psychoanalysis. During the 1950s, the concept experienced a boom, with pivotal works by Hermann (1950), Little (1951), Money-Kyrle (1956), or Racker (1959) being published in rapid succession. Sometime later (especially in german psychoanalysis), works appeared that discussed how actualizations of former relational experiences help constitute the clinical situation and can be understood as they present in the clinical situation ("understanding the scene," Lorenzer, 1970; "action dialog," Klüwer, 1983; "role responsiveness," Sandler, 1976). Also, conceptualizations of an analytic stance of taking in and resonance on the analyst's side play a role here. The latter's relational "offer" consists largely in submitting himself of herself to the experience of crisis, to something that cannot be understood and moreover not be regulated or put into form (see Götzmann & Rüttner, 2017). This also includes the notion that the analyst is not simply present "atmospherically" or as the object of fantasy (yet both plays an important role, e.g., as the "surroundings" for a patient's experience during a session; see, e.g., Schneider, 2005) and reacts accordingly – but also does so on a somatic level, on the level of the body he or she is. The concept of containment (Bion, 1962, p. 145ff.) is not only metaphorically related to a physical body but cannot be thought without the body the analyst is.

Alongside recognizing the importance of embodiment for development and experience (e.g., Leuzinger-Bohleber, Emde & Pfeifer, 2013; Buchholz, 2014), psychoanalysis has come to discuss conceptualizations of somatic countertransference more thoroughly (e.g., Volz-Boers, 2007; Vartzopoulos & Beratis, 2012; Gubb, 2014; from a Jungian perspective: Connolly, 2013; Godsil, 2018). The concept deals with how the analyst directs his or her attention to what "happens" on a somatic level, concerning his or her contact with the patient. Following the understanding of the body one is as discussed earlier we can state that any countertransference affect needs to be under-stood as a somatic phenomenon (see Fuchs, 2018). Yet, in a more narrow meaning, somatic countertransference usually refers to vegetative or muscular processes, pain sensations, an impeded capacity to be attententive, organic mis-sensations, and so on. Zwiebel (1992) describes the analyst's sudden tiredness in relation to defense mechanisms. Zerbe (2019) discusses how unspeakable secrets manifest themselves in the somatic dimension of transference and countertransference.

What happens here is no "countertransference voodoo" by which a patient manipulated, tortured, or aroused us without any physical contact. Rather, what takes place here as unconscious communication (mentioned by Freud, 1912, as communication from unconscious to unconscious) has been described as projective identification, also as a way to conceptualize countertransference more precisely (e.g., Bion, 1959; Ogden, 1979; Frank & Weiß, 2007). Here, as with many other psychoanalytic concepts, the points of view are heterogeneous. I will propose a specific reading and then relate it to somatic countertransference.

The particular value of the concept of projective identification lies in the fact that it refers to more than a mere succession of projective and introjective processes. It refers to a process that on the level of projection already includes the aim for the other to identify with what is projected. Through this, the other can be controlled or function to digest the projected in a way that allows for a subsequent identification. In the case that A projects something in B, we can state that first B identifies himself or herself *with* the projected (in a reflective sense of identifying oneself) and then identifies it *as* something (in a transitive sense of identifying something). Through this, some way of digestion or regulation can take place which then renders it possible for A to take in what was originally projected but has now been made bearable. This is a new identification, now reflexive and potentially transitive. Key to this is that the initial projection is a mental process in A, consisting of a change in the representations of self and object (cf. Zepf, 2006); on an experiential level, something is "deposited" in the representation of the other. Indirectly, namely because a change in self and object representation will also lead to A behaving differently toward B, something of this projection is transmitted to the interpersonal other. The interpersonal digestion relies on the fact that B creates an idea why he or she is treated differently. This is the transition from a being-identified-with to an identifying something. In this, we should not overlook that the unconscious motivation for projective identification is communicating to the other to "do" something with the unregulated in a way that is helpful for the projecting person – but that the process at the same time is marked by something violent and controlling. The other and the projected in him are brought under control, being attacked, etc.

Now, can we resort to this model to conceptually get a hold of somatic countertransference?

First, there is a problem concerning the motive to project in order to (re-) identify with the projected in a digested form. This can hardly be thought of as a process of physical bodily exchange, especially when one takes into account the lack of physical contact between the two persons involved in a psychoanalysis. Yet, we can ask in which way the analyst, via the body he/she is, is reacting psycho-somatically when a patient's projections (as a mental process) result in a different patient behavior toward the analyst – e.g., talking differently or having a different physical posture. This would not come as a surprise since we can easily imagine that the patient being somatically present can influence the "tone" of a session profoundly. So, while we cannot state that a patient deposits something in the analyst (as part of a concrete physical act), we can nonetheless say that the analyst reacts to the unregulated, which is not yet identifiable as something and yet structures the session's tone. He or she reacts as the body he/she is. Through this, he or she co-experiences what it feels like when something is without representational form.

Leikert (2019) also resorts to projective identification (understood as "kinetically encoded communication") in his conceptualization of psychoanalytic treatment technique under the use of the bodily dimension of transference and countertransference. Meaning in a mental sense develops when "the sentient bodily self's subjectivity connects with the perception of a sensual other." For this, a "willingness to incorporate the other within the body one is" (p. 17) is required in the clinical situation. The "encapsulated kinetic engrams" of a body one no longer *is* but merely *has* that are created through inhibition and dissociation and stay separated from experience are supposed to find links regarding a fluid mental form. According to Leikert, this calls for a focus and recognition of bodily sensations and the inclusion of processes of exchange. Here, projective identification is understood as the "transfer of dysfunctional engrams from one body-self to another" (p. 115). The analyst's task is to take "responsibility for his or her own body-self" and to detox it through "systematic attention" (p. 186). Put into other words: Through the analyst's capacity to let himself or herself be used intercorporeally (given the understanding that engrams are separated from the world of representations but not from communication), isolated schemata can find links to experience via a focussing of bodily perception that is initiated by the analyst but conducted together.

In this, we should not forget that "intercorporeal encounters in the clinical field [...] seldomly have the quality of a loving embrace" (p. 17) but have to be understood as an event of crisis. Thought of as projective identification, these processes of exchange are likely to be more intense when the impairment in a patient's mental structure is severe (cf. Goetzmann & Ruettner, 2017). That kind of projective identification in the course of which the analyst at first senses some bodily reaction can be thought of as the expression of searching for and struggling with boundaries on the patient's side. The prominent inclusion of the body one is in this might have to do with an impairment of otherness on a fundamental level. In conceptual terms, projective identification rests on the precondition of a basic separation between the representations of self and object (which renders it plausible why projective identification plays a minor role or is even absent in psychotic disorders; Storck & Stegemann, 2021). The kind of projective identification that leads to bodily phenomena would then be a fundamental one, likely to be unstable, and while some aspects of the mental are warded off from the self, it results in an instantaneous fusional contact. This is a direct way of expellation and ingestion (similar to projective reduplication as described by de Muzan, 1977), a process with constant attempts to establish links and demarcation at the same time because a permeable boundary and a non-dreadful form of emotional touch are not yet thinkable (cf. for thoughts on similar attempts to reach integration Kobylinska-Dehe, 2019).

Level of Interventions II: Interpretations as "Boundary Events"

So far, we are able to understand why there are some dynamics of non-verbal communication and evacuation in somatic countertransference and how these can (and need to) be taken in by the analyst. How can this lead to interventions, and how can a transformative process (cf. Plassmann, 2019; Leikert, 2019) be initiated?

To sum up what has been discussed so far: Phenomena of bodily countertransference can be understood against the background of the dynamics of missing boundaries: Aspects of the inner model of experiencing relationships and relatedness are being communicated on the level of form instead of content. If we modify Freud's words, we can state that the *self* is first and foremost a bodily one (in terms of the body we are), and then bodily countertransference shows how self and object come into contact, e.g., in the dynamics of fusion and in separateness. Also, bodily countertransference can be understood along the line of a "dosage": Something is too much (excitation) or too little (regulation) so that a particular defensive style results which can be understood as a "mandate" to the analyst to help understand and regulate. Working with bodily countertransference aims at the unfolding of a relational space through establishing the experience of contact at a borderline and relatedness despite being different. An interpretation that "works" can thus be understood as a "boundary event" in a multiple sense: It rests on the analyst's experience of crisis which also concerns the body he or she is, and it helps to establish experiencing boundaries – that is, relatedness in the face of psychosomatic difference to the other.

An intervention which rests on this notion should not be trivial, like an analyst simply stating "My arm feels paralyzed" or "I feel tired – any thoughts on that … ?" Bodily countertransference calls for a modulation and the offer to understand what is happening. Of course, interventions always focus the particular material, also the verbal, of a session and clinical event.

The following example shows that:

A 22 years old woman asked for treatment because of symptoms of an irritable bowel and depression. In one session she talks about a visit at her parents'. She wanted to talk to them about how it felt like living on her own for the first time, in a new apartment, but also about how insecure she sometimes felt when it comes to managing„adult" daily life. After the first few minutes her mother took over the conversation and was talking solely, about how she landed an important deal at work and was now putting together a new working group. While talking during the session the patient's voice gradually becomes low and unmodulated, the analysts can hardly hear her until she becomes mute completely. During the resulting silence the analyst feels a heavy dizziness all of a sudden. After one or two minutes he says: "I imagine that there is a part of you that doesn't really know how to show your mother where you are standing." Here, the underlying model of understanding would include that the bodily communication in this session (low voice, communicating through other "channels" than verbal content) marks the question of what belongs to oneself and to the other – and how one's head starts spinning when it is not clear who will take up space talking about what. The body one (no longer) is presents itself also by hardly hearing the patient's voice, it finds a realization in phenomena of transference and countertransference (also, the patient feels the mother does not listen to her, cannot hear her). This shows more clearly and directly what might not be expressed in other ways and has to do with boundaries and contact.

Interpretations and other kinds of intervention stemming from the reflection of bodily countertransference can be categorized similarly to the way we do with interpretations in a more general sense: We might differentiate between analyst-centered and patient-centered interpretations (Steiner, 1993), focus on process interpretations (Plassmann, 2016) or unsaturated interpretations (Will, 2016) – in any case, those interpretations arising out of bodily counter-transference should initiate a process (Storck, 2022).

Conclusion: Mentalized Alterity

The consequences for the theory of treatment technique surely need further elaboration. In this contribution, there was a strong focus on thinking about how to use bodily countertransference as the royal road for establishing contact at a borderline and the experience of being connected and different as elements of an unfolded experiential space for mutual relatedness. If we assume impairments of tolerating otherness which manifest in a struggle with fusional states (whose only alternative seems to be the threat of interpersonal isolation), then we can orientate therapeutic work on focusing the other's otherness in particular or to mentalize the other's alterity. Thus, object representations (and related self-representations) are developing, allowing the experience of connection and relatedness, which no longer comes at the price of having to assimilate but enables the experience of relational intimacy not despite but thanks to intersubjective difference.

Note

1   The author expresses his thanks to Caroline Huss, M.Sc., for her help with the translation.

References

Aisenstein M (2006) The indissociable unity of psyche and soma: A view from the Paris Psychosomatic School. Int J Psychoanal, 87, 667–680.

Alloa E, Bedorf T, Grüny C & Klass TN (2012) (Hg) Leiblichkeit. Tübingen: Mohr Siebeck.

Argelander H (1967) Das Erstinterview in der Psychotherapie. Psyche – Z Psychoanal, 21, 341–368; 429–467; 473–512.

Bion WR (1959) Angriffe auf Verbindungen. In ders (1967) Frühe Vorträge und Schriften mit einem kritischen Kommentar: "Second Thoughts". Frankfurt a.M. 2013: Brandes & Apsel, S. 105–124.

Bion WR (1962) Lernen durch Erfahrung. Frankfurt a.M. 1992: Suhrkamp.

Broschmann D & Fuchs T (2020) Zwischenleiblichkeit in der psychodynamischen Psychotherapie: Ansatz zu einem verkörperten Verständnis von Intersubjektivität. Forum Psychoanal, 36(4), 459–475.

Buchholz MB (2014) Embodiment. Konvergenzen von Kognitionsforschung und analytischer Entwicklungspsychologie. Forum Psychoanal, 30, 109–128.

Connolly AM (2013) Out of the body: Embodiment and its vicissitudes. J Anal Psychol, 58(5), 636–656.

de M'Uzan M (1977) Zur Psychologie der psychosomatisch Kranken. Psyche – Z Psychoanal, 31, 318–332.

Engel GL & Schmale AH (1967) Eine psychoanalytische Theorie der somatischen Störung. Psyche – Z Psychoanal, 23, 241–261.

Fain M (1971) The prelude to fantasmatic life. In Birksted-Breen D, Flanders S & Gibeault A (2010) (Hg) Reading French psychoanalysis. London, New York: Routledge, S. 338–354.

Ferrari AB (2004) From the eclipse of the body to the dawn of thought. London: Free Association Books.

Frank C & Weiß H (2007) (Hg) Projektive Identifizierung. Ein Schlüsselkonzept der psychoanalytischen Therapie. 3. Auflage (2017). Stuttgart: Klett-Cotta.

Freud A (1952) Die Rolle der körperlichen Krankheit im Seelenleben des Kindes. In Die Schriften der Anna Freud, Bd. 4 (S. 1257–1274). München 1980: Kindler.

Freud S (1900) The Interpretation of Dreams. SE 4, 1–625.

Freud S (1912) The Dynamics of Transference. SE XII, 97–108.

Freud S (1916/17) Introductory Lectures on Psycho-Analysis. SE 15, 1–240

Freud S (1917) Mourning and Melancholia. SE XIV, 237–258.

Freud S (1923) The Ego and the Id. SE XIX, 1–66.

Fuchs T (2003) Non-verbale Kommunikation: Phänomenologische, entwicklungs-psychologische und therapeutische Aspekte. Z klin Psychol Psychiat Psychother, 51, 333–345.

Fuchs T (2015) Körper haben oder Leib sein. Gesprächspsychotherapie und Personzentrierte Beratung, 46(3), 147–153.

Fuchs T (2018) Zwischenleibliche Resonanz und Interaffektivität. PDP, 17(4), 211–221.

Godsil G (2018) Residues in the analyst of the patient's symbiotic connection at a somatic level: Unrepresented states in the patient and analyst. J Anal Psychol, 63(1), 6–25.

Goetzmann L & Ruettner B (2017) Veränderungen in der Psychotherapie. Forum Psychoanal, 33, 369–383.

Gubb K (2014) Craving interpretation: A case of somatic countertransference. Brit J Psychother, 30(1), 51–67.

Heimann P (1950) Über die Gegenübertragung. Forum Psychoanal, 12 (1996), 179–184.

Isaacs S (1948) Wesen und Funktion der Phantasie. Psyche – Z Psychoanal, 70 (2016), 530–582.

Karacaoğlan U & Lombardi R (2018) Psychoanalytische Mikroprozesse im Zusammenspiel von Körper und Seele. Jahrb Psychoanal, 76, 93–123.

Klüwer R (1983) Agieren und Mitagieren. Psyche – Z Psychoanal, 37, 828–840.

Kobylinska-Dehe E (2019) Vom Leib zum phantasmatischen Körper – Bewegung, Berührung, Phantasie. Psyche – Z Psychoanal, 73(7), 523–545.

Kohut H (1984) Wie heilt die Psychoanalyse? Frankfurt aM 1987: Suhrkamp.

Kutter P (2001) Affekt und Körper. Neue Akzente der Psychoanalyse. Göttingen: Vandenhoek & Ruprecht.

Küchenhoff J (2010) Die Negativität des Symptoms und die Schwierigkeiten, Nein zu hören. In Küchenhoff J (2013) Der Sinn im Nein und die Gabe des Gesprächs. Psychoanalytisches Verstehen zwischen Philosophie und Klinik. Weilerswist: Velbrück, S. 91–108.

Küchenhoff J (2012) Körper und Sprache. Theoretische und klinische Beiträge zu einem intersubjektiven Verständnis des Körpererlebens. Gießen: Psychosozial.

Küchenhoff J (2019) Intercorporeity and body language: The semiotics of mental suffering expressed through the body. Int J Psychoanal, 100(4), 769–791.

Leikert S (2019) Das sinnliche Selbst. Das Körpergedächtnis in der psychoanalytischen Behandlungstechnik. Frankfurt a. M.: Brandes & Apsel.

Leikert S (2021) Verkapselte Körperengramme und die Traumfunktion – Zur Bearbeitung primärer Abwehrprozesse im Körperselbst. Forum Psychoanal, Online First.

Leuzinger-Bohleber M, Emde RN & Pfeifer R (2013) (Hg) Embodiment. Ein innovatives Konzept für Entwicklungsforschung und Psychoanalyse. Göttingen: Vandenhoek & Ruprecht.

Little M (1951) Gegenübertragung und die Reaktion des Patienten. Forum Psychoanal, 14, 162–175.

Lorenzer A (1970) Sprachzerstörung und Rekonstruktion. Frankfurt a. M.: Suhrkamp.

Luyten P & Fonagy P (2020) Psychodynamic psychotherapy for patients with functional somatic disorders and the road to recovery. Am J Psychother, 73(4), 125–130.

Marty P (1968) Essential depression. In: Birksted-Breen, D.; Flanders, S. & Gibeault, S. (2010). (Hg.): Reading french psychoanalysis. London: Routledge, S. 459–462.

Marty P & de M'Uzan M (1963) Das operative Denken ("Pensée opératoire"). Psyche – Z Psychoanal, 32 (1978), 974–984.

Mcdougall J (1978) Plädoyer für eine gewisse Anormalität. Gießen 2001: Psychosozial.

Mcdougall J (1989) Theater des Körpers. Weinheim: Verlag Internationale Psychoanalyse.

Merleau-Ponty M (1964) Das Sichtbare und das Unsichtbare. München: Fink.

Money-Kyrle R (1956) Normal Gegenübertragung und mögliche Abweichungen. In: Frank C & Weiß H (2013) (Hg) Normale Gegenübertragung und mögliche Abweichungen. Zur Aktualität von R. Money-Kyrles Verständnis des Gegenübertragungsprozesses. 2. Aufl. Frankfurt a.M.: Brandes & Apsel, S. 19–36.

Ogden TH (1979) Die projektive Identifizierung. Forum Psychoanal, 4 (1988), 1–21.

Plassmann R (1993) Organwelten: Grundriß einer analytischen Körperpsychologie. Psyche – Z Psychoanal, 47, 261–282.

Plassmann R (2016) Die Technik der Prozessdeutung. Forum Psychoanal, 32, 443–460.

Plassmann R (2019) Transformative Sprache. Forum Psychoanal, 35, 5–17.

Racker H (1959) Übertragung und Gegenübertragung. Studien zur psychoanalytischen Technik. München, Basel 1988: Ernst Reinhardt.

Sandler J (1976) Gegenübertragung und Bereitschaft zur Rollenübernahme. Psyche – Z Psychoanal, 30, 297–305.

Scharff JM (2010) Die leibliche Dimension in der Psychoanalyse. Frankfurt aM: Brandes & Apsel.

Scharff JM (2021) Psychoanalyse und Zwischenleiblichkeit. Frankfurt aM: Brandes & Apsel.

Schneider G (2005) Vom Zimmer des Analytikers zum inneren Raum des Patienten. In Matejek N & Müller T (Hg) Symbolisierungsstörungen. Göttingen: Vandenhoek & Ruprecht, S. 50–77.

Schultz-Venrath U (2021) Mentalisieren des Körpers. Stuttgart: Klett-Cotta.

Smadja C (2001) The Psychosomatic Paradox. London 2005: Free Association Books.

Steiner J (1993) Orte des seelischen Rückzugs. Stuttgart 1998: Klett-Cotta.

Storck T (2016a) Formen des Andersverstehens. Gießen: Psychosozial.

Storck T (2016b) Psychoanalyse und Psychosomatik. Die leiblichen Grundlagen der Psychodynamik. Stuttgart: Kohlhammer.

Storck T (2018a) Trieb. Grundelemente psychodynamischen Denkens, Band I. Stuttgart: Kohlhammer.

Storck T (2018b) Szenisches Verstehen. In Gumz A & Hörz-Sagstetter S (Hg) Psychodynamische Psychotherapie in der Praxis. Weinheim: Beltz, S. 57–70.

Storck T (2019) Objekte. Grundelemente psychodynamischen Denkens, Band IV. Stuttgart: Kohlhammer.

Storck T (2020a) Verschmelzung oder Isolation – Zum psychodynamischen Dilemma der Objektbeziehung bei psychosomatischen Erkrankungen. Jahrbuch für Kinder- und Jugendlichen-Psychoanalyse, Band 9: Psychosomatik – Sadomasochismus – Trauma. Frankfurt a.M.: Brandes & Apsel, S. 184–202.

Storck T (2020b) Übertragung. Grundelemente psychodynamischen Denkens, Band V. Stuttgart: Kohlhammer.

Storck T (2021a) Die Schmerzerfahrung als Suche nach Grenzen und Kontakt zum Anderen. In Eusterschule A & Benini E (Hg) Kritik(en) des Leidens. Berlin: Neofelis.

Storck, T. (2021c) Mentalisierung und die Pariser Schule der Psychosomatik. Forum Psychoanal, 37(1), 87–97.

Storck, T. (2021d) Die Gegenübertragungs-Jukebox. Über eine Idee, wichtige Grundlagen der psychoanalytischen Haltung anschaulich zu machen. Psyche – Z Psychoanal, 75(12), 1074–1178.

Storck T (2022) Deutung. Grundelemente psychodynamischen Denkens, Band VIII. Stuttgart: Kohlhammer.

Storck T & Brauner F (2021) Körpergefühl. Gießen: Psychosozial.

Storck T & Stegemann D (2021) Psychoanalytische Konzepte in der Psychosenbehandlung. Stuttgart: Kohlhammer.

Taubner S (2015) Konzept Mentalisieren: Eine Einführung in Forschung und Praxis. Gießen: Psychosozial.

Taubner S, Fonagy P & Bateman A (2019) Mentalisierungsbasierte Therapie. Göttingen: Hogrefe.

Theunissen M (1977) Der Andere. Studien zur Sozialontologie der Gegenwart. Berlin u.a.: de Gruyter.

Vartzopoulos I & Beratis S (2012) Bodily manifestations in the psychoanalytic process. Psychoanal Q, 81(3), 657–681.

Volz-Boers U (2007) Psychoanalyse mit Leib und Seele: Körperliche Gegenübertragung als Zugang zu nicht symbolisierter Erfahrung und neuer Repräsentanzenbildung. In Geißler P & Heisterkamp G (Hg) Psychoanalyse der Lebensbewegungen. Zum körperlichen Geschehen in der Psychoanalytischen Therapie – ein Lehrbuch. Berlin: Springer, S. 39–58.

von Rad M (1983) Alexithymie. Empirische Untersuchungen zur Diagnostik und Therapie psychosomatisch Kranker. Berlin, Heidelberg, New York: Springer.

Warsitz RP (2004) Der Andere im Ich. Antlitz – Antwort - Verantwortung. Psyche – Z Psychoanal, 58, 783–810.

Will H (2016) Ungesättigte und gesättigte Deutungen. Psyche – Z Psychoanal, 70, 2–23.

Zepf S (2006) Allgemeine Psychoanalytische Neurosenlehre, Psychosomatik und Sozialpsychologie. Band 1. Gießen: Psychosozial.

Zerbe KJ (2019) The secret life of secrets: Deleterious psychosomatic effects on Patient and Analyst. J Amer Psychoanal Assn, 67(1), 185–214.

Zwiebel R (1992) Der Schlaf des Analytikers. Die Müdigkeitsreaktion in der Gegenübertragung. 3. Auflage (2010). Stuttgart: Klett-Cotta.

Contributors

Christophe Dejours is a physician, psychiatrist, and psychoanalyst, a full member of the Association Psychanalytique de France, a full member of the Institut de Psychosomatique-Pierre Marty (Paris), and a president of the Scientific Council of the Fondation Jean Laplanche-Institut de France. He is Chair Emeritus of Psychoanalysis and Healthwork at the Conservatoire National des Arts et Métiers in Paris and Professor Emeritus of the University of Paris-Nanterre. His research interests lie in psychosomatics, the psychoanalytic theory of sexuality and Laplanche's theory of generalized seduction, theory and metapsychology of the body, and clinical and work psychodynamics. His recent publications include (2001) *Le Corps d'abord – Corps biologique, corps érotique et sens moral*; (2012) *Psychopathogien der Arbeit. Klinische Fallstudien* (Psychopathologies of Work. Clinical Case Studies); and (2010) *Körper und Sexualität in der Psychosomatik* (Body and Sexuality in Psychosomatics).

Lutz Goetzmann, Prof. Dr. med., psychoanalyst (SGPsa/IPV), presently in psychoanalytic practice in Berlin. Medical studies in Homburg/Saar, psychoanalytic training at the Freud Institute Zurich, and habilitation at the University Hospital Zurich. 2011–2020 Chief Physician at the Clinic for Psychosomatic Medicine and Psychotherapy, Bad Segeberg. Since 2014, he has been an APL Professor at the University of Lübeck. Co-founder of the Institute for Philosophy, Psychoanalysis, and Cultural Studies (IPPK) and co-editor of the journal *Y – Zeitschrift für Atopisches Denken*. Numerous publications on psychoanalytic psychosomatics. His recent publications include (2020) *Gamma Elements as Protomental Representations: Suggestions for Expanding W. R. Bion's Model of Elements*; and Goetzmann, L., Siegel, A., Ruettner, B. (2020): *On the Axis of Psychosomatic Totality.*

Ewa Kobylinska-Dehe, Dipl.-Psych., M.A., Dr. Phil., professor of theoretical psychoanalysis and philosophy at the Polish Academy of Sciences, co-founder and vice director of the Centre for Psychoanalytic Thought in Warsaw, and co-editor of the journal *Wunderblock*. Psychoanalysis and philosophy, psychoanalyst and supervisor (IPA, FPI), teaching analyst (Anna Freud Institute), honorary member of the Polish Psychoanalytic Association. Works on hermeneutics, methodology of cultural studies, psychoanalysis in cultural modernity, psychoanalysis and phenomenology, corporeality, and transgenerational transmission of trauma. Her recent publications include (2021) Psychoanalyse zwischen Hermeneutik und Neurowissenschaften. In: *Wie Phönix aus der Asche. Psychoanalyse in Nachkriegspolen* (Psychoanalysis between Hermeneutics and Neuroscience. In: Like a Phoenix from the Ashes. Psychoanalysis in post-war Poland); (2022) *Nur der Fremde kann uns retten. Freud und das Unheimliche* (Only the stranger can save us. Freud and the uncanny); (2022) Ist die Welt aus den Fugen geraten? Psychoanalyse für eine überforderte Gesellschaft. In: *"Zeitdiagnosen!?"* (Has the world gone off the rails? Psychoanalysis for an overstrained society. In: "Diagnostics of our time!?"); and (2023) *Thinking Cure. Jewish Psychoanalyst Aleberta Szalita, from Warsaw to New York*, Routledge.

Sebastian Leikert, Dr. en Psychanalyse (Paris), Dipl. Psych., Psychoanalyst (DGPT), is an affiliated member of the DPV. Private practice in Saarbrücken. Lecturer and training analyst at the Institute for Psychoanalysis and Psychotherapy Heidelberg (DGPT), lecturer and training analyst at the Saarland Institute for Psychoanalysis and Psychotherapy (DPG), Chairman of the German Society for Psychoanalysis and Music (DGPM). Member of the Editorial Board of *The International Journal of Psychoanalysis* and *The Psychoanalytic Quarterly*. His recent publications include (2019) *Das sinnliche Selbst – Das Körpergedächtnis in der psychoanalytischen Behandlungstechnik* (The Sensual Self – Body Memory in Psychoanalytic Treatment Techniques); (2021) *Encapsulated Body Engrams and Somatic Narration – Integrating Body Memory into Psychoanalytic Technique*; (2023a) *Unrepresented states and the bodily unconscious*; and (2023c) *Falling, Primitive Separation and Encapsulated Body Engrams – Working through a Bodily Encoded Unconscious Syndrome*.

Riccardo Lombardi, Dr. med., is a psychiatrist and psychoanalyst, and practices in Rome. He is a member of the International Psychoanalytic Association, training analyst and supervisor of the Italian Psychoanalytic Society, and a member of the editorial board of the *Journal of the American Psychoanalytic Association* and *The International Journal of Psychoanalysis* and the advisory board of the Yearbook of Psychoanalysis. His recent Publications include (2015) *Formless Infinity: Clinical Exploration of Matte Blanco* and (2017) *Bion and Body-Mind Dissociation in Psychoanalysis: Development after Bion*.

Reinhard Plassmann, Prof. Dr. med., is a specialist in psychosomatic medicine and psychotherapy, a specialist in neurology and psychiatry, a DPV training and control analyst, and an EMDR therapist. He worked for many years in inpatient psychotherapy, most recently as Medical Director of the Psychotherapeutic Center in Bad Mergentheim, until 2014 as a Professor at the University of Kassel, since 2014 as a Professor at the International Psychoanalytic University Berlin IPU. He furthermore has a private practice in Tübingen. His main research interests include modern emotion research and its consequences for treatment techniques. His recent publications include (2019) *Psychotherapie der Emotionen. Die Bedeutung von Emotionen für die Entstehung und Behandlung von Krankheiten* (The Psychotherapy of Emotions. The Importance of Emotions for the Development and Treatment of Diseases); and (2021) *Das gefühlte Selbst. Emotionen und seelisches Wachstum in der Psychotherapie* (The Felt Self). Emotions and Psychological Growth in Psychotherapy.

Jörg M. Scharff, Dr. phil., Dipl.-Psych., psychoanalyst (DPV/IPA). Since 1980 in private practice. Training at Pro Familia, at the Anna Freud Institute in Frankfurt, and as a lecturer and training analyst at the Frankfurt Psychoanalytic Institute. Publications, among others, in *Psyche* on psycho-analytically oriented counseling, on staging interaction, on the relationship between inner and outer factors in psychoanalytic theory, on psychoanalytic treatment techniques, and on the musical aspects of analytic dialog. In recent years, he has focused on "interbody" states in the psychoanalytic situation. His recent publications include (2010) *Die leibliche Dimension in der Psychoanalyse* (The Bodily Dimension in Psychoanalysis); (2013) together with S. Leikert: *Korrespondenzen und Resonanzen. Psychoanalyse und Musik im Dialog* (Correspondences and Resonances. Psychoanalysis and Music in Dialog); and (2020) *Psychoanalyse und Zwischenleiblichkeit. Klinisch-propädeutisches Seminar* (Psychoanalysis and Interbody States. A Clinical-Propaedeutic Seminar).

Ulrich Schultz-Venrath, Prof. Dr. med., is a specialist in psychosomatics and psychotherapy (DGPM) and neurology (DGN), a psychoanalyst (DPV, IPA, DGPT), and a group training analyst (D3G, IGAM, EFPP, GASI) in his own private practice in Cologne. He is a professor of Psychosomatics and Psychotherapy at the University of Witten/Herdecke and was Chief Physician of the Clinic for Psychiatry, Psychotherapy, and Psychosomatics of the EVK Bergisch Gladbach from 1999 to 2019. He has contributed to numerous publications on group analysis and the history of psychoanalysis. He is a spokesman for the Editors of the journal *Gruppenpsychotherapie und Gruppendynamik – Zeitschrift zur Theorie der Gruppenanalyse* and Spokesman for the Advisory Board for Science and Research of the D3G as well as Editor of the series *Mentalisieren in Klinik und Praxis*. His recent publications include (2021) *Mentalisieren des Körpers* (Mentalizing the Body); and (2022) *Mentalisieren – Psychotherapien wirksam gestalten*/(Mentalizing – Designing Psychotherapies Effectively).

Timo Storck, Dipl. Psych., Dr. phil., psychological psychotherapist and psychoanalyst (DPV, IPA, DGPT), professor of clinical psychology and psychotherapy at the Psychological University of Berlin. Research focus: psychoanalytic conceptual research and methodology, theory of illness (psychosomatics, compulsion, psychosis), film psychoanalysis, and concept-comparative psychotherapy research. His recent publications include (2018–2022) *Basic Elements of Psychodynamic Thinking* (eight volumes); and (2021) *Body Feeling* (together with Felix Brauner).

Ursula Volz-Boers, Dr. med., psychoanalyst (DPV/IPA) and group analyst, Dr. of psychosomatic medicine and psychotherapy, Dr. of neurology and psychiatry, training analyst of the DPV/IPA and supervisor in the Cologne Psychoanalytic Institute of the DPV (Psychoanalytische Arbeitsgemeinschaft Köln-Düsseldorf e.V.), as well as attachment analyst. She has her own practice in Kamp-Lintfor/Niederrhein. She has published on the theory and technique of psychoanalytic treatment of early traumatization, physical counter-transference as access to unsymbolized experience, and new representation formation. Her recent publications include (2007) Psychoanalyse mit Leib und Seele: Körperliche Gegenübertragung als Zugang zu nicht symbolisierter Erfahrung und neuer Repräsentanzenbildung (Psychoanalysis with Body and Soul: Bodily Countertransference as Access to Nonsymbolized Experience and New Representational Formation). In P. Geißler & G. Heisterkamp (Eds.): *Psychoanalyse der Lebensbewegungen. Zum körperlichen Geschehen in der psychoanalytischen Therapie – ein Lehrbuch* (Psychoanalysis of Life Movements. On Bodily Events in Psychoanalytic Therapy – A Textbook); and (2016) Resonanz im Körper des Analytikers. Das Konzept der sensorisch-intuitiven Haltung (Resonance in the Analyst's Body. The Concept of the Sensory-Intuitive Stance). In S. WalzPawlita, B. Unruh & B. Janta, B. (Eds.): *Körper-Sprachen* (Body Languages).

Index